Look Younger than Your Age
Healthy Life

Mary Milionis

Acknowledgements

Writing this book has always been a dream for me. It was something I wanted to do once in a lifetime. It would never have come into existence without the support of my family, friends, and dearest clients.

I have gained enormous knowledge and insight into my work from my clients. My education also had a major role in my over 40-year career as an esthetician. It is what I have shared in this book. I have shared all my experiences with you in this book. I must confess that I am thankful to my wonderful clients for their encouraging response over the years. I couldn't have done this without you.

Skincare, for me, has been not only my job but also my favorite hobby. This is also one of the reasons why I wanted to write this book to help others understand its importance and overall impact on our health. Successful skincare treatment has been one of the most rewarding accomplishments of my life. In this book, I have taken the time to explain several ways to have healthy and younger-looking skin along with a healthy lifestyle.

I want to thank my son George Milionis for helping me edit this book and providing me with the right legal counsel. Thank-you to my daughter Effie Milionis Verducci for all her technical assistance throughout the time I was writing my book. A special thank-you to my husband, Konstantin Milionis, for your endless love and support. And a thank-you to the rest of my loving and supportive family, who helped me make my book successful.

I want to thank Dr. Sears for providing me with all his vitamins' information and sharing his studies that helped me over the years to understand the importance of having a healthy body and younger-looking skin. Also, I want to thank Dr. Sobel for providing me with education. I have learned a lot from him over the years about life cells and skincare treatment.

I finally found the time to grab a pen and shape my story into words. This is my attempt to trap all my experiences and learning in a single book. This book is not only about understanding the skin and skincare routine but also about helping others lead a healthy life along with having younger-looking skin. This combination, for me at least, has been a key factor in keeping my skin healthy over the years.

In the end, I want to thank everyone who is taking the time to read and understand my book and follow up with a healthy lifestyle. I assure you if you use the information provided in this book rightly, you will have clearer and younger-looking skin.

Look good. It feels good!

About the Author
Meet Mary

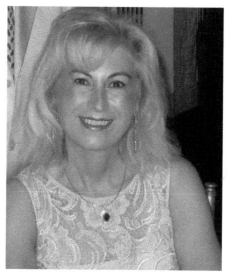

Mary Milionis is the founder of Biotherapy Esthetics, a skincare products company. She is also the founder and previous owner of the Esthetique European Skin Care Clinic in San Mateo, California. As a licensed esthetician, she has more than 40 years of skincare experience, having worked with thousands of clients to solve their most sophisticated skincare challenges. Aside from her love for healthy skin, she is passionate about healthy living regimes, too. She lives in California with her husband and has two grown-up children and five grandkids.

In this book, Mary Milionis draws upon her over 40 years in the skincare industry as an experienced and dedicated esthetician. After learning and mastering the art of skincare, including the effects of a proper skincare regime and high-quality products, she decided to elevate her passion for skincare and become a licensed paramedical esthetician in 1996.

Having been educated in Greece, Switzerland, and the United States, Mary continued her education and pursued extensive education focusing on skincare and proper skincare treatment. She has additional training in anti-aging treatments, chemical peels, and exfoliation techniques, including ultrasonic peels. Over the past three decades, she has treated all skin types and conditions using the most advanced skincare products and systems available on the market today.

As the previous owner of the Esthetique European Skin Care Clinic in the Bay Area, Mary has seen over 1,000 patients. As a result of the extensive patient studies and treatments over this time, she developed two private skincare lines of Esthetique Skin Care and Biotherapy Esthetics.

After this extensive experience, practicing skincare treatment and helping countless patients with acne problems and other skincare issues, she now shares her deep knowledge in this book for the benefit of readers who are passionate about healthy skin.

Preface

Since I can remember, I have always been asked, *"What does it take to keep my skin look so healthy and young?"* I want to answer this question once and for all.

Not only my past clients ask this but also my family, friends, and acquaintances who are curious about my skincare routine. I usually tell them that **what you do** will have a drastic effect on **how** their skin looks. Yes, it really does matter how you treat your skin. Not only is it your largest organ, but it also needs as much (or perhaps more) attention as anything else in your body. Proper skincare doesn't have as much to do with skin color, genetics, and exposure to the sun as you might think.

After so many years of living my mantra of good skincare, I thought it was time to put pen to paper and share my experiences – both good and bad – about what daily routines and simple lifestyle changes can do for your skin. I hope this journey is as enjoyable for you as it is for me to share.

In this book, we will explore some basic concepts that cover healthy skin. These concepts will build upon each other, including skincare regimen for morning and night, using skincare products *correctly* with high-quality ingredients, protecting your skin from the sun, eating healthy and drinking plenty of water, avoiding alcohol and smoking or being around others who smoke, exercising at least three times per week, and so much more. We will draw upon each one of these concepts individually for you to understand their impact on your skin.

Remember, everything I just mentioned matters, as healthy skin does not happen overnight, and it also doesn't happen with any miraculous cure (at least none that we know of). I love taking care of my skin and I think it shows that.

So, come join me on this journey, so I can share with you all my secrets to younger and healthier skin.

Contents

Page Left Blank Intentionally

Introduction

Who doesn't like to look younger than their age and live a healthy life? No matter how much we emphasize being young at heart, looking young equally matters for everyone. Women often take it as a compliment when someone tells them that *you look way more youthful than your age*. They blush and smile about it throughout the day. Trust me; there is nothing wrong with wanting to look younger than your age.

Looking young has a lot to do with self-confidence. Men get attracted to women who appear younger than their age. Looking young boosts confidence because when you look good, you feel good. Consequently, you begin to obsess over things like your skin and weight, which is yet another healthy habit.

Unfortunately, women tend to age and look older earlier than men. There can be numerous reasons behind that, including stress resulting in acne, obesity due to pregnancy, and many others. We will discuss each of them in detail throughout this book. Moreover, we are all so caught up in our lives that we often forget to take care of ourselves, especially our skin. I am here to remind you that you must take good care of yourself. I will leave this book at your table to keep reminding you how vital it is to take care of your skin to look and feel young.

Looking young has a direct link with a healthy body and skin. Sadly, our skin is something that we pay the least attention to. Therefore, I need you to stop for a while and ask yourself, *do you have a skincare routine or you just fall asleep every night, not caring about what is on your skin?*

In addition to so many benefits, a healthy skincare routine can help you establish other healthy habits that you always wanted to build. It gives you the motivation you always needed. It is certain that if you can create this one habit, you can create other healthy habits, too. They may include oral care and hair and scalp care routines. When you do them all, you look and feel good.

Are you persuaded enough to gift yourself a skincare routine? The next question you may ask is, *how do I do that? How do I take care of my skin?* Well, these are just two of dozens of questions I get asked from my clients on a regular basis. What are the things I can practice to take care of my skin? What are the best products to use? How should I use the recommended products? What do I need to put on my skin at home? How do we build a healthy lifestyle on the basis of everyday routine? What are the best products for my skin type? How to stay healthy and not overweight? Do vitamins have anything to do with the health of my skin? Is the sun bad for our skin? Does smoking affect our skin? How about drinking alcohol? What is the impact of drinking alcohol on our skin? Does it put our skin in danger? There were many such questions I came across during my career as an esthetician. Well, relax! I am here to clear all your doubts and help you develop a routine.[1]

"You look way younger than your age. What's the secret?" It is the one question I often hear from my clients, friends, family, and physicians. Even my doctors ask me a lot of questions about what I do in my everyday life that I look so young. I visited three of my physicians at different times for annual checkup, and all three of my doctors at different times said the same thing, *"You are way healthier than any other women of your age. Will you please take the*

---

[1] *7 REASONS WHY YOUR SKINCARE ROUTINE IS IMPORTANT*
https://www.stockpilingmoms.com/7-reasons-why-your-skin-care-routine-is-important/

time and explain what do you do to keep yourself young and healthy? What's the secret?"

If you are wondering the same, here's a piece of good news for you. I am here to share that secret with you. This cannot be a coincidence, right? Not to overrate my health and skin, but these are only a few examples of the things I get to hear on a regular basis. Therefore, through this book, I want to educate people, especially women, on living a healthy life, looking younger, and staying happy. I want them to get the same satisfaction that I get when I hear such kind words. I aim to write this book that will help others add to their beauty and reach a point where they wish to live a long and healthy life.

For those of you still wondering who I am, my name is Mary Milionis, and I have always been passionate about skincare. I have more than 40 years of skincare experience, having worked with thousands of past clients to solve their most complex skincare challenges. Aside from my love for healthy skincare, I am passionate about healthy living regimes.

In regard to my personal life, I live in California with my husband. We are blessed to have two grown-up children.

Besides my two children, I am also blessed with five grandkids.

I have been a part of the skincare industry for more than 40 years and have worked as a dedicated esthetician. In case this word is entirely new for you or you don't know who an esthetician is, let me explain it to you. An esthetician attends a separate program and is licensed to provide specific skin condition treatment, custom skincare routine recommendations, and skin mapping.

I have been to various places to receive the education and knowledge I have today. I received my training from Greece, Switzerland, and the United States. I never let anything come between my passion and myself. This book is also the by-product of that same passion. I am so glad that I am capable of writing it. I have continued to gain knowledge and pursued extensive education related to skincare and maintaining ideal skin. Moreover, I have received additional education and training in anti-aging treatment, chemical peels, and exfoliation techniques, including ultrasonic peels.

After learning and mastering the art of skincare and proper skincare regime and dealing with high-quality products, I decided to elevate my passion for skincare. I became a licensed paramedical esthetician in 1996. This was the best gift I could give myself to enable me to help others make their skin better.

When I see others' skin healing, it gives me satisfaction beyond explanation. I have treated all skin types and conditions in the past three years with the help of the most advanced skincare products and systems available on the market.

My Experiences

I have treated thousands of patients as I was the founder and previous owner of the Esthetique European Skin Care Clinic in San Mateo, California. I treated my clients for 27 years with different types of skin treatment, including collagen treatment, life cells treatment from Dr. Sobel, a supplier from Canada, in 1989. It was huge back then in the beauty industry. Its impact on the skin cells' life was also amazing. Now it has become stem cell therapy, which is something quite similar today in the beauty industry. The treatments I provided were huge on glycolic acid, including peels, Vitamin-C treatment, youth light treatment, ironic treatment, and my regular weekly facials. Believe me; they were all so effective that I had a lot of clientele to treat and manage. There were many things I learned from my experience as an esthetician, stories I came across, and lives I touched. I was treating almost a thousand repeat clients, and the satisfaction I was getting back in return can never be described in words. It was a pleasant feeling at the end of the day.

I am proud to announce that with the help of years of education and experience in the field, I have developed two private skincare product lines of Esthetique Skin Care and Biotherapy Esthetics. I would have never been able to do this without my extensive patient studies and treatments over a long time. After this extensive experience of practicing skincare treatment and helping countless patients with acne skin problems and skincare issues, I have now innovated a private skincare line for all skin types with robust, effective, and therapeutic ingredients. My product line also has a sub-specialty focused on dry or sensitive mature skin with wrinkles. Every product has been tried, tested in the labs, and hand-chosen by myself. These skincare tools can be used to make your skin healthier and look years younger.

Why Am I Writing This Book?

I have learned that people neglect skincare due to a lack of time and knowledge, unaware of the dangers that lie ahead. Believe it or not, this is my dream book. I aim to educate people about things they did not know or cared about throughout this book. I want to help people look younger than their age since it is the key to a happy and healthy life.

You will learn how to build habits that result in healthy skin and a healthy lifestyle in the chapters ahead. You will also learn about how to choose the right skincare routine for yourself and the right products and look and feel good.

This book is not only for older women. It is for everyone wishing to change their routine and take care of their skin. I want to help people of all ages and direct them to the right method to skincare and healthy life as a daily routine.

I will not let this experience stay limited to only external factors and products. Haven't you heard the statement, "*You are what you eat?*" Everything you put in your body affects you and, eventually, your skin. So, we will take all the possible factors under consideration, and I will educate you about the things you can eat and exercises you can do to keep your skin and body healthy.

They say that it doesn't matter how you look, but let me tell you that your appearance matters at the end of the day. Your face is the first thing people notice about you, and you do get judged by your appearance.No matter if it is a job interview or finding your significant other, how you present yourself matters. I need you to realize that your appearance has a lot to do with your skin. Many people put themselves and their skin in danger by choosing the wrong and cheap products and living an unhealthy lifestyle. I am here to extract that negative attitude and lifestyle from you and fill you with all the positives that I know.

As I said earlier, it is not only my past clients who ask this but also family, friends, and acquaintances who are just curious about skin. My answers are according to my education and how I took control of my lifestyle. Of course, it did not happen overnight. Things take time, but it is never too late.

I usually tell them what you do will have a drastic effect on how your skin looks. Yes, it really does matter how you treat your skin. Your skin is not only your largest organ, but it also needs as much and even more attention as any other part of your body. A proper skincare routine doesn't have as much to do with skin color, genetics, and exposure to the sun as you might think.

Fast food is another enemy of the skin. You will learn about all the other enemies as you walk my journey in your imagination via this book. It will work as a portal that contains all the information and things you need to know about your skin. The goal of this book is to build a bridge for everyone that leads to a healthy lifestyle.

Things You Should Do

In this book, we will explore some basic concepts that cover healthy skin. These concepts will build upon each other. Here is a brief introduction to them, so you have a clear idea of what you will be learning throughout this book.

Skincare Regimen for Morning and Night

What type of in-home skin routine do you have? What you apply to your face, neck, chest, legs, and other parts of your body does matter more than you might think. While some people approach skincare with a once-a-day cleanser in the morning or night or both, there is more that should be done to make the pores clean, create elasticity, and attain an overall healthy skin.

Use Skincare Products Correctly with High-Quality Ingredients

Spending big bucks on the most expensive products is not the solution. Instead, there are both key ingredients as well as key interactions of skincare products that together yield cleaner skin, which allows your skin to thrive. The by-product is healthier and younger-looking skin.

Protect Your Skin from the Sun

Yes, apply that sunblock even on rainy days. Stay out of direct interaction with the sun when possible. These are rules you already know, of course. However, there are additional protocols for dealing with the sun in addition to the sunblock and shading. One key concept here is that UV radiation damages not only the first layer of the skin but also the second and even third layers. So, there are ways to keep all these layers protected from the sun, not only with sunscreen but also with hydration, eating right, and avoiding smoking.

Eat Healthy and Drink Plenty of Water

This is not as simple as it sounds, of course. Coming from Europe, we did not have all the temptations that I find here. There was no fast food option for me as I grew up. But that doesn't mean those options are not around now, and frankly, I do indulge in them but only once in a while. We will cover what fast food does to your body and skin. More importantly, we will cover what happens when you eat foods that are natural, low in fat, high in antioxidants, and high in key minerals and vitamins. We will also talk about how important it is to drink water. You may already know it, but we will look at it from a skincare perspective. It's not only good for your body, but it also prepares your skin for *defense mode*, for fighting off toxins, UV, smoke, scratches, and even makes you bounce back from a long night. I could not emphasize more. However, there is much more to be discovered.

Don't Smoke or Be around Others Who Smoke

Although you do not smoke, the effects of second-hand smoking are equally damaging to the collagen in your first and second layers of skin. Think about smoke as the neutralizer to the above rules (healthy eating, avoiding the sun, and staying hydrated) because smoke can tighten the first layer of your skin.

If you are a smoker, it will also limit blood flow, which damages your skin and collagen. The effects of smoking on the look and feel of your skin can be terrible over time. So, we will discuss methods to keep your skin protected from the smoke.

Exercise at Least 3 Times per Week

Exercising has always been good for both the body and the skin. In fact, the effects of exercise on the skin are well known. For example, one study found that when your heart beats faster, muscles pump out more of a certain protein, which in turn powers skin cells to act younger. In fact, over time, exercising can make your skin look and feel about 25 years younger at the microscopic level.[2]

All of the steps mentioned above matter as healthy skin does not happen overnight, and there is no miraculous cure to it (at least none that we know of). I love taking care of my skin and I believe it appears.

---

[2]*See study from McMaster University in Ontario:*
https://www.ncbi.nlm.nih.gov/pmc/articles/PMC4531076/

So, are you ready to attain your dream skin and dream life, where you are happy in your skin and confident about how you look? I am sure you are because nobody wants to live a life where they have to doubt constantly whether they are looking good enough? Come join me on this journey, so I can share with you all my secrets to younger and healthier skin. I want to discard all the doubts from your life and create a world where people do not start to feel old way before their time.

It is true that when you love yourself, only then can you allow others to love you. When you do that, you can keep yourself healthy as well as others. When you feel good about yourself, only then can you make others feel good about themselves. Remember, negatives only bring negatives. You cannot expect positivity out of someone who is negative about their own self all the time. Not liking yourself can be traumatic for many, so it is vital that you care about yourself enough not to let yourself fall into that black hole.

Healthy life matters and it can only be created by eating healthy food, exercise routine, wearing sunblock, and avoiding unnecessary medications. Yes, what matters the most is what's inside a person, but why not opt for the best life when you can? Why choose to live a life where you don't care about how you appear because you do not feel good about your appearance anyway. It's time that you add up to your beauty and feel good about yourself inside out. It's time that you give your life a pause and choose to love yourself enough. When you care about healthy skin, you will eventually develop a healthier lifestyle, with a healthy-looking body and face.

"When you can feel good about yourself, it carries into everyday life. If you can look in the mirror and like yourself, that's the greatest feeling in the world." **Dick Bryant**

Chapter 1- What Does It Take to Look Younger than Your Age?

Hello there! I am happy you decided to proceed and make efforts to live inside your dream skin. I am sure after reading the introductory chapter, you will know well how vital it is to take care of your skin. I am glad that you are willing to learn the secret of looking younger than your age. Looking and feeling young are two things that everyone wants, and there is nothing wrong with it. Let's begin with this beautiful quote:

"Aging is a fact of life. Looking your age is not." **-Dr. Howard Murad**

There is nothing to be ashamed about wanting to look younger than your age. You have the right to feel good about yourself. Many times, people age faster and start to look older than their age. They lose self-confidence and feel helpless at the same time. They think there is no way they can get back their old skin, which is not true. So, it's okay if you want to make efforts to look younger than your age, and it's alright if you are serious about it.

Your skin takes quite a bashing from your environment throughout your life since it protects you from all the harmful elements you are surrounded with, such as the sun and the harmful UV rays it exhibits. Therefore, it is no surprise why the appearance of our skin keeps changing with time.

The first step to looking good is taking care of your skin. If you want to reverse your biological clock of aging and look years younger than your actual age, it's time to make changes to your lifestyle. In this book, we will look at several aspects of life that must be changed and habits that have a healthier impact on your skin. Remember, you are what you eat, and the lifestyle you adopt today will determine how you will look a few years later.

Remember, it's never too late to start taking care of your body's largest organ that works overtime to protect you and your skin. Whatever you are going through in life appears on your skin. Whether it is stress, tiredness, unhappiness, an unhealthy lifestyle, or happiness, your skin says it all. It automatically glows when you are living a healthy life full of happiness and fades away when you are sad or upset. The skin is the organ that keeps the whole body together.

So, what does it take to look younger than your age? Your lifestyle has a huge role to play here since it directly impacts your skin and body. Your diet, toxins in your environment, stress level, whether you smoke or not, how much you sleep, and how much you exercise all have an impact on your skin. Here are a few things you need to take care of to look younger and healthier.

Eat Healthy Food

A poor diet is always bad news for your skin. Looking beautiful and glowing inside out mostly come from within your body. We often hear the phrase, *you are what you eat.* It is the most authentic thing you can make yourself believe in. Whatever you put inside your body will determine how your skin appears and how well you look overall. Whatever you put inside your body later shows on your epidermis, your skin.

Hence, eating healthy is crucial to the human body. Some foods can harm it, while others can help it heal. A poor diet can affect your skin in multiple ways, causing dryness, dehydration, premature aging, clogged pores, and puffiness. It may even contribute to acne in some people. Hence, you must be very careful about your food choice and must avoid eating too much fast food, sodas, alcohol, pizza, starch, tin-food, pasteurized food, French fries, salad dressings, and butter bread. In fact, a better substitute for butter bread is olive oil on the bread roll. It tastes even better and is definitely healthier.

The solution to healthy, glowing skin, if you don't have acne, is to follow a balanced diet that is rich in protective nutrients such as vitamins, minerals, and dietary fiber. However, following a low-GI diet will help you maintain a healthy body and skin if you also have acne issues. In case you don't know what GI is, the Glycemic Index (GI) is a number assigned to food from 0 to 100, with pure glucose arbitrarily given the value of 100. It represents the relative rise in the blood glucose level two hours after consuming that food.[3]

Remember, a healthy diet is also important for your appearance. Eat fresh fruits and vegetables as much as you

---

[3]*Glycemic index*
https://en.wikipedia.org/wiki/Glycemic_index

can. Other foods that you can consume include unsifted grains and cereals, yogurt and cheese, low-fat milk, fish, eggs, and lean meat. Try to consume monounsaturated fats and oils, which will make sure your body gets all the vitamins, minerals, and omega fatty acids it needs for flawless skin and good overall health. These small yet effective changes in your eating habits will benefit you and your skin a lot in the long run.

"Being healthy is something I learned from a very young age. Looking after yourself on the inside helps with your energy, makes your skin glow, and changes your whole outlook on life." **-Phoebe Tonkin**

Go Out and Exercise

Gather all your nerves and the motivation you have when you go to the gym and start exercising. In fact, you can exercise however you want and at any time of the day. You only have to get moving if you want to improve your skin's health. Sweating helps clear out pores and flush out impurities from the skin. Exercise is yet another part of your life, which is incredibly vital for your health. The exercises I find the healthiest are inexpensive and easy to perform.

These include outdoor running, walking, or even if you are taking exercise classes, making sure they're outdoors. The fresher air you inhale, the better it is for your health. The most effective exercises are walking, jacking, or running outside, in my personal opinion.

Outdoor activities help oxygen reach the brain and the lungs, which works as a booster for your heart. When your heart functions better, it enables your brain to think better and faster. It sometimes helps find the answers you need much more comfortably. Therefore, everyone needs a piece of outdoor activity, at least once a day, for a short time.

It also helps us get over sorrow and pain. Our biggest problems can be resolved just by spending some time close to nature. When people run into the ups and downs of life, the best doctor to the matter is giving yourself a break by walking or running, by employing in outdoor activities.

Stay Out of the Sun

When you go out for a walk or a run, it should be in the evening when the sun rays are at their lowest power. Protect your skin from interacting directly with the sun as much as you can. Although we all need a little bit of sunshine every once in a while to boost vitamin D level, our skin can get damaged by the harsh rays of the sun.

Ultraviolet (UV) radiation causes loss of elasticity, wrinkles, sun spots, and premature aging. These changes begin to show at an early age in some people. Therefore, you need to be ruthless in protecting your skin from the sun. Always wear sunblock. I recommend SPF #30 for the face and SPF #50 for the body. SPF #30 can be applied to the body as well, but SPF #50 should never be applied to the face. A higher number can block your skin's pores, so stick to SPF #30 when it comes to your face.

Moreover, always cover up, wear a hat, reapply sunscreen, and wear UV-protective sunglasses when you go out in the sun, even on cloudy days. They may seem small at a time, but if you see closely how bad sun rays can affect your skin in a short time, you will never go out in the sun.

Drink Plenty of Water

Water is probably the best remedy for healthy skin and overall appearance. Usually, the person who always carries a water bottle and drinks plenty of water has a fair complexion and soft skin. In case you don't know, our skin contains plenty of water and needs a standardized hydration level to keep it healthy, glowing, soft, and smooth. What happens if you drink less water? You will automatically experience dry skin and some acne problems. Science suggests that people can gain amazing benefits from drinking one gallon of water a day. It keeps the skin cells hydrated and moisturized, which, in turn, protects the skin from pimples, blemishes, darkness, and wrinkles. Believe me, your skin can glow without the highlighter if you drink enough water, which also has plenty of other health benefits (except you will have to bear with a lot of peeing). Women need to drink at least three liters of water a day to keep their bodies hydrated and skin glowing and reach the ideal level of fitness.[4]

Get Your Beauty Sleep

Your skin needs at least eight hours of sleep for the renewal of the skin cells. Not getting the required amount of sleep results in a lackluster appearance and breakdown of collagen. This, in turn, will highlight even minor skin

---

[4]*Does Drinking Water Really Make Your Skin Glow?*
https://thecoldestwater.com/does-drinking-water-really-make-your-skin-glow/

imperfections you may have, making you look older than you should. Moreover, lack of sleep may cause dark circles under your eyes. They are a result of dilated blood vessels, which makes you look tired and old. Also, you must be careful not to sleep too much, or the skin-cell breakdown may be encouraged. Sleeping for longer hours than normal can also make the body lose flexibility.

Get Body Massages

If possible, routinely take body massages once or twice a month. They are greatly beneficial to the body and the skin. A full body massage helps remove dead skin cells from your body, resulting in the reduction of dullness and bringing fresh skin to the surface. It can also help regenerate new tissues and cells, reducing the appearance of scars and stretch marks. Oil massage moisturizes the body.

Moreover, a body massage helps improve blood circulation running to the arteries, helps muscles get stronger, and helps the heart run at a regulated speed. It is a perfect remedy for people suffering from high blood pressure. Body massages also circulate cells to our body due to which our body keeps a large number of cells without being active after a certain age. A good massage helps the body and soul to relax and revive from stress, tension, and external pressure. It relaxes the whole body and makes you look younger than your age. So, ladies, I recommend that you spend some time at the spa, for it brings youthfulness to your body. Eventually, it translates into your face.

It Will Help If You Stop Stressing

We don't realize it often, but stress can severely affect our entire body, including our hair, nails, and skin. It gives birth to a chemical as a response in your body that makes skin more sensitive and reactive.

Did you know that stress leads to the production of a hormone called cortisol? This hormone commands your body to create more sebum, the oil found in your skin. As a result, your skin may become oily or spotty. It can also make it harder for skin problems to heal. Of course, stress can also worsen existing skin conditions such as eczema and psoriasis. It can also cause other types of skin rashes such as hives and trigger a flare-up of lymph fevers.

What makes you think that stressing out is any good for you or will it solve any of your problems? Since it is an unavoidable part of our life, what matters the most is how you handle it. You need to be patient and give your body and mind some time to heal.[5]

Avoid Unnecessary Medication

You must realize that all medications cause side effects. For instance, almost 5% of the population can be allergic to some sort of antibiotics. One of the common reactions is skin rashes. In fact, some antibiotics interact with alcohol negatively and can cause severe reactions like skin flushing, acne, upset stomach, fast or irregular heartbeat, headache, or drowsiness, which is why I say to avoid unnecessary medication as much as you can. They can prove to be unhealthy for both your body and skin.[6]

Avoid Alcohol as Much as You Can

Drinking alcohol is yet another bad habit that you need to get rid of. It's never a part of a healthy diet, so you should

---

[5]Your lifestyle and your skin
https://www.health24.com/Lifestyle/Perfect-Skin/Natural-Beauty/Your-lifestyle-and-your-skin-20140115

[6]Medicines and side effects
https://www.betterhealth.vic.gov.au/health/ConditionsAndTreatments/medicines-and-side-effects

already know about its ill effects. Drinking alcohol does not only produce another adverse reaction to your skin, but it also destroys brain cells and causes memory loss. Moreover, it is as bad as smoking and affects the liver and lungs.

Nevertheless, its impact on the skin shows first in the form of wrinkles, dryness, blemishes, and brown spots. It is essential to know that when we grow old and reach the age of above 50, our body stops replacing the cells being destroyed by alcohol. The body's recuperation of cells gets reduced with age, increasing the impact of alcohol intake.

This is also the reason why we lose memory, energy, and youthfulness in old age. Some people develop depression quite easily. So, why take such a significant health risk? It's better to take necessary precautions today than regretting tomorrow.

Get a Facial Massage Done Every Month

Nothing can compare to the feeling you get when you glide your fingers over your face and feel that soft and milky skin. Facials are hugely beneficial to the skin. Having them done once a month can surely make a difference. They remove the dead cells from your epidermis and allow it to breathe. They penetrate into the third layer of the skin. They also work best for a daily skincare regime.

I am not only saying things because they are apparently effective, but I have also seen the results with my eyes. Over the years, I have shown my clients the beauty of monthly facial routine or every two weeks of treatment of exfoliation to the skin. The expiration of their skin's beauty was amazing to witness.

I feel sorry for the women who do not have the opportunity to try and take facials often, but there is one thing they can do - home facials. There were times when my co-estheticians and I used to finish our working day and practice facial treatment on each other. It was one of our best times that also helped us enhance our beauty. So, if you cannot go to a professional to get it done, home facials are good to go, as long as you are using quality products.

Facials are vital because they help reduce stress, relieve psychological distress, prevent aging, exfoliate your skin, open up all the pores, cleanse, tighten, restore, and detoxify your skin. They also help eliminate under-eye bags, dark circles, whiteheads, and blackheads. Your face needs to be pampered, even if you do not have blemishes, hyperpigmentation, severe acne, or any other significant problem. So, the next time you feel that facials are not necessary, read this again.

How to Do Facial at Home

In case you are too naïve to do home facials, relax. I will share some simple and easy steps that lead to great skin. One of the great and effective skincare lines is the biotherapyesthetics.com (Do not forget to do a patch test first). All you have to do is follow these steps.

Step # 1: The first step is to massage your face with a cleanser. Use a sponge to remove it from the skin. Wiping it off with warm water is always the best step.

Step # 2: The second step is to apply the toner (lotion) to finish cleansing the pores.

Step # 3: The third step is to apply glycolic acid, which you will find especially significant in your facial treatment.

Step # 4: The fourth step is to use a clay mask. Silk amino mask is one of the best masks available on the market. You will also find it at the biotherapy esthetics line. Apply the mask on top of the glycolic acid all over your face, neck, and delicate area.

Leave the mask on for a good ten minutes. Afterward, remove it with a washcloth and warm water. Follow up with toner again. Apply the eye cream, face moisturizer, and sunblock if it's a day. Always remember, it is greatly beneficial to give a facial to yourself during nighttime. After the treatment, apply a good amount of super firming nighttime cream. Again, you will find it in the biotherapy skincare line.

The next day, your skin will feel silky soft and youthful as if you have got new skin all over again. Let me give you a little introduction to my skincare line. Biotherapy Esthetics Skincare line is an amazingly effective component to add to your daily routine. You will see the difference in your skin right after using these products for the first time. It took me a long time to develop this incredible line for both women's and men's skin beauty, for they deserve equal care. Every piece has been studied, tried, and tested in the labs to produce the absolute best results.

In case you are thinking of buying some products for yourself, the best-sellers are the eye cream, oxygen cleanser, and super firming nighttime cream. They all have amazing results. Not to brag, but I am speaking from experience. My skincare line is for all skin types and works more effectively for mature skin. So, now you know what you need to do next. For me, skincare is not only my hobby but also a passion. When I help women with their beauty needs, I feel accomplished by the end of the day.

Consistency Is the Key!

If you started a new diet and didn't see results in a day, you wouldn't throw in the towel. The same goes for skincare. Remember, consistency is the key.

Trends come and go, but some things should always remain the same, especially when it comes to your skincare regimen. I often come across people who complain about their skin's results, yet they are very inconsistent when it comes to following the daily routines. They do not realize that consistency is imperative when it comes down to making the most of a cream, supplement, or oil.

We are talking about building habits here. So, if you are not consistent, how in the world are you going to possibly do it? If you do not believe in your skincare routine and do not make specific changes to your lifestyle, you won't be able to make a difference to your skin. Therefore, it is extremely important that you continually take care of your skin. You will soon witness the changes in yourself. So, what are you waiting for? Start the process of looking younger than your age today. I promise you, you will not regret it.

Always remember the following key points.

Results Take Time

You simply cannot expect a miracle to happen overnight and see better-looking skin straight away. In fact, you generally have to wait a few weeks and sometimes a month to see the results. So be patient.

Maintain Good Skin

Consistency extends your skin's life. Think of it in the same way as brushing your teeth. You do it every day to ensure you maintain good oral health. Your teeth begin to deteriorate when you don't do it over time, and they fall out if you stop taking care of them. You don't want the same to happen with your skin, right? So, maintain good skin by all means.

It Only Takes a Few Minutes

While it may take a few weeks to see the results of your skincare routine, it only takes a few minutes of your day to take care of and maintain your skin. Yes, all it takes is a few minutes to be consistent in your skincare routine.

Just like you make time to work out for an hour, take some time to do skincare. Keep reminding yourself that it only takes a few minutes and you will find yourself doing it more often.

It Gets Easier with Time

Once you build a lifestyle, things will get easier. You will not have to think twice about doing your skincare routine. It may take some time to build new habits and change the old ones, but you should not give up. Keep your eyes on your goal - looking and feeling good.[7]

It's okay to forget sometimes. What's not okay is making it a habit. So, make sure you focus on building the right habits. With this message, this chapter comes to an end.

---

[7] *Why consistency is key in a skincare regime*
https://my.lumitylife.com/why-consistency-is-key-in-a-skincare-regime/

Happy Younger Looking Skin Life! But hold on, there's more to come.

Chapter 2- Skincare

Like every other part of your body, your skin also requires attention and special care. This is probably the best time to be alive as there are so many effective skincare products for you to try. However, if you are not careful, those products can be quite harmful in the long run.

Every skincare product is a package of hope. You excitedly start using it, wondering whether it will decrease those dark circles or magically make those dark spots disappear. How long will it take? We often become impatient. It all depends on the products you choose and how severe is your skin's condition. It is good that you think about resolving your skin problems. However, before you get into the process of making your skin better, let us first learn about how our skin ages and the layers that it contains.

The outermost layer of the skin is called the epidermis. It consists of five major layers. The primary function of the epidermis is to act like the body's safety shield to the environment, temperature, and radiation exposure and provide feedback to the brain. It consists of small flat cells that get smaller and flatter as they approach the surface of the skin.

Gradually, the cells on the surface become keratin – a dead protein – as they reach the outermost layer called the stratum corneum. This process of *keratinization* takes three to four weeks. The epidermis also houses nerve endings and melanocytes that produce melanin – the primary agent that gives skin its color. Melanocytes are isolated at the stratum Basale layer of Caucasians, but they extend into the dermis in the skin of darker persons. Carotene is yet another pigment (yellow-orange) found in the stratum corneum and fatty areas of the dermis.

Factors Affecting Your Skin
UVA/UVB Light and Skin Aging

Aging causes the skin to become thinner and lose its elasticity. It also slows down the natural cycle of skin replacement. A controlled study was done to ascertain the difference in skin changes due to aging and sun damage. Skin roughness mostly increases due to chronological aging, whereas loss of skin elasticity was found to be predominately caused by damage from the sun.

The exposure to ultraviolet radiation triggers a repair response, causing the epidermis to thicken. It also increases melanin production, degenerates collagen, and forms irregular elastin fibers and dilated twisted blood vessels. UVA light causes lipid peroxidation, and UVB light causes mutagenic and carcinogenic effects. UV light induces enzymes that degrade skin collagen.

Heat

Heat excites the sweat glands, which secrete fluids to cool the skin. Excessive heat damages the epidermis and causes loss of water, nitrogen, protein, and minerals. Showering or bathing in hot water can also cause skin damage.

Smoking and Alcohol

Smoking constricts and damages the arteries that supply nutrients necessary for the health and growth of the skin. This, in turn, reduces the rate of new cell production and subsequent turnover rate of the skin. Consequently, your skin becomes less elastic and drier with deeper fine lines. In essence, smokers wear their faces longer than nonsmokers. Whereas, alcohol constricts the arteries that supply nutrients to the skin. Moreover, people who consume lots of alcohol usually do not get proper vitamins and minerals.

Nutritional Impacts and Skin Health

For your skin to be healthy, it is necessary to ensure that appropriate vitamins are supplied to your body through diet. Vitamin deficiencies most often exhibit their initial symptoms via the skin. The deficiency of important vitamins can contribute to dryness, scaling, skin discoloration, or even lesions in some cases. One should ensure that they have an adequate intake of vitamins, so their body does not have to face any kind of deficiency.

The Impact of Skincare Routine

Let's break down the skincare products into moisturizers, serums, cleansers, and masks and examine how long it would take for an individual product to have an effect on fine lines, hyperpigmentation, dark circles, dry skin, and acne. Let's see how they affect our skin.

Moisturizers

A moisturizer can produce immediate (and pleasing) effects, or it can do nothing at all, depending on what you are hoping to get out of it. Some moisturizers have ingredients like hyaluronic acid. They offer immediate improvements, but the effects would not last long. However, many of the latest moisturizers include ceramides, which are naturally occurring lipids in our skin. They improve the skin barrier, so they would help with dryness. Results can be seen in as little as a week, and they'll extend over your natural skin cycle. This means permanent improvements.

The best way to select a moisturizer is by looking for ingredients like retinol and vitamin C. These components have the best science behind them, working to diminish the appearance of fine lines. Using a product with one or both of these ingredients will yield results anywhere from several weeks to months, but you must stay consistent to see the results.

There is not much that a moisturizer will do to address hyperpigmentation or rosacea. But if you are using a prescription cream, which will usually be caffeine-based to help with the restriction of blood vessels, you'll start to see improvement in as little as two to three days. For a minor acne inflammation, an over-the-counter product with benzoyl peroxide will take effect in a day or two. While, a prescription medication will likely take care of it in one application. Moisturizers rarely have any lightening effect on the dark circles.

Serums

Serums are the opposite of moisturizers. They contain active ingredients, but they produce long-lasting results. If you are using a serum with alpha hydroxy acid or vitamin C, you will have to wait longer to see results. If you are using it to improve skin smoothness, diminish fine lines, repair dryness, or address dark spots, and give it at least four to six weeks to see lasting results.

The best ingredient to look for is vitamin C. It helps repair sun damage along with other benefits. Its effects are both long-lasting and immediate.

Cleansers

Here's the thing about cleansers. They don't have much of an effect on any particular skin issue, but using the wrong one could create a host of problems. Hence, it is essential to pick the right one. Switching to a proper, gentler cleanser without irritating botanical ingredients or too much fragrance will yield a noticeable improvement in the texture and appearance of your skin in only a couple of weeks. However, you must understand that a cleanser is not a magic potion. It will not wash your acne away.

Pro tip: Cleansers often contain surfactants that are necessary to clean the skin. However, they can cause irritation or rashes. Toners may also contain alcohol or acids such as alpha hydroxy acid (AHA), which can cause skin problems in some people. So be incredibly careful in selecting one for yourself. Remember, always check the ingredients.

Masks

You will seldom see an immediate improvement in the tone and texture of your skin after a single use of a mask, no matter the purpose. A mask is designed to take off the stratum corneum of the skin (the dead top layer of skin). It will clamp down on your pores, which is why it gives an instant glow. For long-lasting results, you will have to use a mask once a week with an active ingredient, like salicylic acid, for acne. It will result in noticeable skin improvement within six weeks. Consistency is the key here.

Pro tip: Applying masks involves the use of the manual application, that too of chemicals on the skin. It often results in exfoliation of the upper skin surface. Mild irritation is inevitable, but severe skin inflammation like dermatitis can also occur. Don't worry if such a thing happens. Apply lots of ice cubes and again, beware of what suits your skin and what doesn't. Do a patch test, always.[8]

Setup a Skincare Routine – What Products to Use

The skin is the largest organ of the body. When it comes to the skin of your face, it is very sensitive and extremely vulnerable to the environment. Factors like the condition of the weather, wind, dust, heat, and cold can surely have an effect on your skin. As I said earlier, it is essential to protect your skin from the sun. Good SPF creams help prevent and erase brown spots from the face if you use them every day.

Many people ask me what my skincare routine is and what products they should use to keep their skin healthy and young as I do. As an esthetician, I would like you to

---

[8]This is how long it will take for your skincare routine to work
https://globalnews.ca/news/4113894/skincare-routine-effects-time/

approach an incredibly easy and pleasant skincare regiment as a daily routine. The important point is to ensure that you don't become lazy and stop doing it after a while. A complicated skincare routine can result in you turning your face away from it, so keep it simple. Of course, we all need solid and quality skincare products. Here's what you can do to take care of your facial skin.

Step # 1: Apply a potent oxidizing face cleanser in the morning and at night. Remove it from the face using a sponge or soft washable cloth.

Step # 2: Use a scrub with glycolic acid in it and wash your skin with this scrub twice a week.

Step # 3: Use a toner (lotion). It helps to close the pores and maintain their correct size as well. Apply it with a piece of cotton, if possible.

Step # 4: Apply eye cream around the eyes, between eyebrows and upper lip area in the morning and at night. A night cream is especially important for the face. I recommend applying a layer of extraordinarily strong glycolic acid before the night cream. It will do the work overnight and make the products even more effective. When I use this method, my skin feels quite silky the next morning.

Step # 5: Use sunblock as much as you can. Apply it to your skin on all days, whether sunny or cloudy, even if you plan to stay inside.

Step # 6: Do not forget to take the right vitamins. Your body produces skin, bone, and muscle every single day. It sends nerve signals skipping along thousands of miles of brain and body pathways. It churns out rich red blood that carries nutrients and oxygen to all body parts. It also formulates chemical messengers that shuttle from one organ to another, issuing the instructions that help sustain your life.

However, to do all this, your body requires some raw materials. These include at least 30 vitamins, including vitamin C, D, and K, minerals, and other dietary components that your body needs but cannot manufacture on its own in a sufficient amount. Vitamins and minerals perform hundreds of roles in the body. They help heal wounds, shore up bones, and bolster your immune system. They also convert food into energy and repair cellular damage. Therefore, it is important that you take care of the vitamin intake of your immune system.

Tada! You have successfully set up a highly effective skincare routine. Now, stick to it as if it's an obligation, and you will soon see the results.

Pay Attention to Your Neck

Your daily skincare routine should not end at your chin. You must consider taking care of your neck. Our neck is the most delicate skin area and needs additional care. It is also the area that ages first because it has many pores, and its skin is quite sensitive. But we pay the least attention to it. This is why I need you to make sure you use the most effective products in this area. Sometimes, no products are available on the market, specifically for the neck. In that case, it's okay to use your night cream. At least pay attention to it, and you will see a wonderful response.

Normalize Using Skin Masks

What is a skin mask and why do we need to use it at least once a week? A mask exfoliates the dead cells of the epidermis. Basically, it offers deep cleansing of the pores. Before you apply a clay mask, it is vital to apply glycolic acid first and follow up with a thick layer of the clay mask, including your neck. Leave it on the skin for at least 10 minutes. Wash it off with warm water using a washcloth. Apply a toner and eye cream right after washing it off if it's daytime. If it's night already, apply night cream.

Always avoid applying makeup right after washing your face for a good half hour. For best results, use the mask during nighttime. The next morning, your skin will look like you had a facial from a professional salon the night before.

Benefits of Taking Care of Your Skin

You may not think much about this or perhaps you avoid thinking about it, but the reality is that taking care of your skin is vital. Taking care now ensures that you will not have to worry about it worsening over time. If you do not take the necessary steps for your skin, you can face many skin issues like acne. It can often make a person feel incredibly unattractive, and they are always at a risk of losing self-confidence. I don't want you to be one of them.

How you treat your skin and what you feed it determine your skin's health, just like other parts of the body. A healthy skincare routine ensures that your skin has the nutrition it needs to heal and repair itself, maintain the finest functionality, and hold on to youthful flexibility.

However, taking care of your skin goes beyond just looking and feeling beautiful. Here are several reasons why one must take care of their skin.

Healthy Skin Is Vital to a Healthy Body

To understand the importance of a skincare routine, you first need to realize why it is essential to take care of your skin. Whether you accept it or not, your skin is your body's first line of resistance against every possible threat present in your surroundings. Healthy skin provides a barrier that prevents millions or even billions of pathogens from entering your body. These pathogens can cause infection, disease, and discomfort to your body.[9]

Our Skin Sheds Itself Every Day

Did you know that your skin cells shed almost every second all the time? It means that the healthy skin you have today could be gone by tomorrow. Isn't it enough to

---

[9]*Why Is Skin Care So Important?*
https://www.halecosmeceuticals.com/why-is-skin-care-so-important/

motivate you to develop a good skincare routine? An effective routine can help prevent acne, treat wrinkles, and keep your skin at its best.

We All Have Different Skin Types

Maybe, you have a friend who does not have any skincare routine, but they still have great skin. Perhaps, you think that you don't need a skin routine, but you need to know that every skin type is different. Our skin may require more attention and care than the person sitting next to us. It makes daily skincare routine essential for staying young.

Beautiful Skin Is a Lifelong Process

If you want flawless skin thirty years from now, start working for it today. The choices you make today are going to have an impact on your life throughout. Beautiful skin is a lifelong process. You can only enjoy it if you build a care routine. A healthy skincare routine today will help you maintain beautiful skin in the future. Similarly, not caring for your skin will have a negative impact and affect its overall appearance in the future.

Prevention Is Easier than Cure

Preventing your skin from potential problems now is easier than trying to fix skin issues in the future. It takes less time to involve yourself in a skincare routine than to see dermatologists every other day or address complicated skin issues down the line. To avoid such problems, you should stop neglecting your skin in the first place.

A Skincare Routine Saves You Money

When you develop a healthy skincare routine, you avoid many skin-related problems that are already there or may occur in the future. If you don't want to deal with acne scars, skin discoloration, deep wrinkles, or other skin problems, make time to take care of your skin just like you make time to check your Facebook. This will prevent costly treatment requirements and medicines in the future. A healthy skincare routine now will prevent future trips to a dermatologist or plastic surgeon.

When You Look Good, You Feel Good

Shrink-wrap protects what's inside. Similarly, your skin is your body's wrapper and plays the role of its protector. It becomes your identity and helps recognize you among other people. Your skin tone, texture, and how it wraps around your features are different than everyone else. Everything combined creates the appearance that makes you who you are. Don't you want your presence to look perfect?

When you are confident about your skin, you feel good within and become confident about yourself. Remember, your face is the first thing that people see without even knowing you. It automatically creates the first impression in others' minds. When someone looks at you, don't you want to make it worthwhile? A daily skincare routine can help you achieve all of this, boosting your confidence at the same time. So why not have one?

I hope by now, you are confident enough to select products on your own and are quite aware of the results if you set up a skincare routine.

Pro tip: Happy skin is the key ingredient to a happy life.

Chapter 3- The Sun

We all grow up hearing not to go out in the sun, bare skin. It can harm your skin. But we never take it seriously. Now, as an aesthetician, I realize how essential it is to protect your skin from the sun. If you search for it now, you will find thousands of studies that discuss how harmful sun rays are for the skin, but I speak from experience.

Exposing your skin to the sun is not a joke. You do not need those harmful UV rays damaging your skin. During my career as an aesthetician, I came across many patients who helped me understand how sun rays can severely affect our skin. There are two types of UV radiations: Ultraviolet A (UVA) and Ultraviolet B (UVB). The difference between the two is that UVA can pass through the glass, whereas UVB cannot pass through such mediums. However, they can both cause different skin diseases. Hence, you must protect yourself from both.

Here are a few reasons why you should protect your skin from the bright sun.

Sunburn

At some point in life, we all get sunburns. But do you know that severely excessive exposure to the sun rays can damage your skin? It becomes red and its texture weakens. The skin starts to peel after the initial sunburn. It even feels irritated, and this can go on for weeks. This is when you can tell that you have a sunburn, and if you are not careful, it can lead to painful blisters.

One of the most fundamental reasons why you must wear sunscreen all summer long is to avoid sunburn. Hence, if you plan on being outside all day, you must continuously apply sunscreen at least every two hours. It becomes incredibly important that you apply sunblock, especially if you know you will be out from 10 A.M. to 4 P.M. This is the time when the sun is the highest in the sky and can produce extreme sunburn. If you plan on swimming, go for a waterproof sunscreen. Reapply sunscreen when you are out of water. It may seem you are overprotective, but trust me, your skin will be gracious.

Skin Cancer

There are millions of people who are diagnosed with cancer every year in the United States. Skin cancer is one of the most prominent variations of cancer in the country. One of the best ways you can avoid getting skin cancer is by putting on sunscreen when you go outside. The UV radiation from the sun reaches your skin and causes damage, which can later turn into a malignant tumor. It is also the reason why you must apply sunscreen all over, as it can form anywhere on your exposed body. Ensure you cover everything, including your face, arms, neck, legs, and torso, if you know they will be exposed to the sun.

While it is incredibly vital to wear sunscreen throughout summers, you should wear it all year long. The sun is going to rise in the winters too. So chances are, you can still get a sunburn and you are still at risk for getting skin cancer over time. Therefore, do not season-bound this crucial element of your daily care routine.

Premature Aging

Some UV rays penetrate deep into the skin and can damage it severely, which leads to premature aging. It is also why most people face saggy skin and wrinkles sooner than they would like. Other common signs of premature aging include redness, sunspots, and tanned skin. It is better to avoid them in the first place, although there are treatments to prevent them.

According to research, people who wear sunscreen are less likely to develop signs of aging at an early age. Sunshine damages essential components like collagen and elastin. So, to keep your skin looking younger and healthier, you must get your hands on the best sunscreen that you can find.

Sunspots and Hyperpigmentation

Generally, sunburn is temporary. The skin becomes red for a little while and then it clears up after a week or so. However, some problems stick around for a little longer. Sunspots and hyperpigmentation are among them. They indicate that skin tissues have taken on the damage. So, if your skin is already damaged, it is alarming for you. You must immediately take action since you do not want to feed your skin any more fatigue.

Tanned Skin

Many people like to have tanned summer skin. What they do not know is that tanned skin often showcases injured skin. To protect our skin from UV radiation, our body has a protection mechanism. Our body can then get to work on repairing the skin, and it goes back to being fair. Nevertheless, this process is not healthy for you. Excessive tanning will lead to sunburn, meaning your tan will eventually peel.

While lying out in the sun is not good for your skin, you also need to be careful of the tanning beds. Many studies show they are harmful to the skin. It is high time that you realize how tanning is overrated and that your health is more important than looking great.

Skin Condition You Already Have Can Worsen

If your skin is already suffering, you do not need to add to your troubles by exposing it to UV radiation. For instance, many Americans suffer from varicose veins. They usually form in the legs and can damage the blood vessels when left in the sunlight for long periods. Sunlight breaks down the collagen in the legs and penetrates down into the skin's blood vessels. This is why you must put sunscreen on because it prevents blemishes, blotchiness, and red veins.

We all want our skin to remain healthy. There are certain things you can do if you are not happy with your skin for some reason, but remember that sunlight is not going to heal your skin anyway. You should avoid going out in the sun as much as you can.

I cannot emphasize more how vital it is to protect your skin from the sun. The more you take this advice, the better it will be for your skin.[10]

Sun Protection Tips

Here are a few safety measures that you should take to protect your skin from sunlight.

Limit Sun Exposure

As I mentioned earlier, the harmful sunrays are the most intense between 10 A.M. and 4 P.M., so be extra careful

---

[10]8 IMPORTANT REASONS TO PROTECT YOUR SKIN IN THE SUN
https://www.timelessha.com/blogs/news/8-important-reasons-to-protect-your-skin-in-the-sun

while going outside during these hours. If it's essential to go out, then practice the shadow rule. If your shadow is shorter than you, you should find shade. Always keep children younger than six months inside the shade and completely covered.

The UV Index Deserves Your Attention

This numbered scale measures how damaging exposure to the sun will be on any particular day. It is often included in the weather report. People should try to stay indoors when the index is ten or higher.

Be Careful around Reflective Surfaces

Water, sand, and snow reflect the damaging rays of the sun and increase your risk of getting sunburned.

Wear Protective Clothing and Sunglasses

By protective clothing, I mean wear clothes with long pants and long sleeves and a hat that shades the neck, face, and ears. Compared to white or loosely woven fabrics, dark clothes with tightly woven fabric block more sunlight. Search for clothes made with special sun-protective materials for added protection. When it comes to sunglasses, make sure they have 99% to 100% UV absorption.

Beware of Medication's Side Effects

Some medications can make you extra vulnerable to the sun. They may include anti-inflammatories, specific types of antibiotics, medications for blood pressure, some types of chemotherapy, and antifungals.

Avoid Recreational Sunbathing

Avoid tanning beds, sun lamps, or tanning salons as much as you can. Focus on having healthy skin instead of attractive skin.[11]

Use Sunscreen

Most importantly, you must use sunscreen. Damage from the sun rays happens over time, which makes it essential to apply sunscreen every day, even on cloudy days. Here are a few tips for applying sunscreen.

---

[11]Protecting Your Skin from the Sun
https://www.cancer.net/navigating-cancer-care/prevention-and-healthy-living/protecting-your-skin-sun

Use Sunscreen with Broad-Spectrum Protection

Choose a broad-spectrum sunscreen that protects against both UVA and UVB radiations. Make sure it has a sun protection factor (SPF) of 30 or higher and it is water-resistant. Other types of sunscreen will not protect against skin cancer, although they may help prevent sunburn. When compared to each other, SPF sunburn protection is not proportional to the SPF number. For instance, SPF 30 does not provide double the protection of SPF 15. Above SPF 50, studies have found that the additional protection benefits are minimal. So, don't stress about looking for a sunblock higher than that number. Also, do not forget to use a lip balm or lipstick that contains sunscreen with an SPF of at least 30.

Use the Right Amount of Sunscreen

Apply a generous layer. Do not skimp. Instead of rubbing it, smooth it down. According to the American Academy of Dermatology, you must use one ounce of sunscreen, equivalent to the amount of a full shot glass. It is then enough to cover your entire body, including your ears, neck, face, the tops of your feet, and your scalp if you are bald or have thinning hair to achieve the ideal level of protection.

Apply (and reapply) Sunscreen Properly

According to the American Academy of Dermatology, apply sunscreen to dry skin 15 to 30 minutes before going out in the sun and every time you come out of the water or sweat. The guidelines also suggest that regardless of its SPF number, reapply sunscreen generously at least every two to three hours, even if the product is labeled *all-day*.

Apply under Makeup

Suppose you wait to apply sunscreen until you hit the beach. In that case, you may already be perspiring, and moisture makes sunscreens less effective. Therefore, women should apply sunscreen under makeup as well.

Never Expose Babies Younger than 6 Months to Sunscreen or the Sun Rays

According to the American Academy of Pediatrics and American Cancer Society, infants should be completely protected from the sun, especially when they are younger than six months. Since a baby's skin is too sensitive for sunscreen, it is not a viable solution. If you need to be outside with a baby, try to cover them entirely in protective clothing and put on a solid hat that also covers their face and neck.[12]

What Is SPF?

We have been talking about SPF for so long. Let me help you understand this term better. SPF, or Sun Protection Factor, is a measure of how well a sunscreen will protect your skin from UVB rays, the kind of radiation that causes sunburn, damages skin, and can contribute to skin cancer. These rays are known to damage the epidermis and other outer layers of the skin. These are also the layers where the most common and dangerous forms of skin cancer may develop.

Therefore, it is quite crucial to use the right amount of SPF according to your skin type. If you burn after being 20 minutes in the sun, SPF 30 protects for about 10 hours, assuming that you use it correctly. However, the wavelength and intensity of UVB rays differ throughout the day,

---

[12]Why sun protection is important
https://www.reidhealth.org/blog/why-sun-protection-is-important

depending on the location. But that calculation does not apply to UVA rays.[13]

Important Tips

Typically, if your skin starts to burn after being 10 minutes in the sun, applying an SPF 15 sunscreen will allow you to stay in the sun for approximately 150 minutes without burning (a factor of 15 times longer). This is a rough estimate that depends on the intensity of sunlight, the amount of sunscreen used, and the skin type. SPF is actually a measure of protection from the amount of UVB exposure. It is not meant to help you determine the duration of exposure.

Many experts recommend using a minimum SPF sunscreen of 15 for best protection, applying the proper amount (2mg/cm^2 of the skin or about one ounce for full body coverage), and reapplying it every two hours.

Most people use ¼ to ½ of the amount required and hence under-apply sunscreens. Only a square root of the SPF can

---

[13]What Does SPF Stand For?
https://www.consumerreports.org/cro/magazine/2015/05/what-does-spf-stand-for/index.htm#:~:text=SPF%20(sun%20protection%20factor)%20is,ultraviolet%20(UV)%20B%20rays.&text=Assuming%20you%20use%20it%20correctly,protects%20for%20about%2010%20hours

be attained by using half the required amount of sunscreen. So, a half application of an SPF 30 sunscreen only provides an effective SPF of 5.5. Moreover, the SPF (Sun Protection Factor) scale is not linear.

- SPF 15 blocks 93% of UVB rays

- SPF 30 blocks 97% of UVB rays

- SPF 50 blocks 98% of UVB rays

Therefore, one way of looking at this is that SPF 30 sunscreen only gives you 4% more protection than SPF 15 sunscreen. Another way of looking at it is:

- SPF 15 (93% protection) allows 7 out of 100 photons.

- SPF 30 (97% protection) allows 3 out of 100 photons.

So, an SPF 30 will block half the radiation that an SPF 15 would let through to your skin, while you may not be doubling your level of protection this way.

Why Not Use a High Sun Protection Factor?

Sunscreens with really high SPFs do not offer any greater protection than SPF 30. No matter if it's SPF 75 or SPF 100, a higher number does not matter. A higher number only misleads people into thinking that it will provide greater protection, but that is not the case.

Moreover, the UVA protection should be at least 1/3 of the UVB protection in order to have broad-spectrum protection. Higher SPF sunscreens usually offer far greater UVB than UVA protection, thus offering a false sense of full protection.[14]

Chemical vs. Mineral Sunscreens

There are two kinds of sunscreen; chemical, which tends to go to the skin easier; and mineral, which is often difficult to rub in. They both differ in their functionalities. Both of these reduce the risk of skin cancer and sunburn and are known to reduce short and long-term damage.

---

[14]WHAT IS SPF SUNSCREEN?
https://www.badgerbalm.com/s-30-what-is-spf-sunscreen-sun-protection-factor.aspx

The primary difference between the two is that chemical sunscreens absorb the UV light, while physical or mineral sunscreen acts more like a shield, deflecting harmful rays from the sun. The common ingredients in chemical or conventional sunscreens include avobenzone, oxybenzone, octocrylene, octisalate, octinoxate, and homosalate. Chemical sunscreens are easy to apply because of their constituents.

On the other hand, mineral sunscreens contain zinc oxide or titanium oxide. It often feels like sticking to the skin. These are becoming more popular in the U.S. because people have started to worry about their bodies absorbing chemical sunscreens' ingredients. There is a possibility that you can absorb a small amount of mineral sunscreen, but it is unlikely if we study how they work. They sit on top of your skin, deflecting the sun rays, and can be washed off with water or sweat easily.

These are all the things that you must know about SPF and its functionality. I hope by now, you know how important it is to wear sunscreen and keep your skin covered.

What Products to Use?

There sure are many brands that you can count on. However, the Biotherapy Esthetics Skin Care products are worth a try. Every product available on my website is tried and tested and hand-chosen by myself. There is a variety of products on my website to choose from. They can help protect your skin and also work as a sunscreen for you.

The science behind skincare products has come a long way. But there is still no such thing as an instant fix. You need to give it some time to reap the benefits. All you need to do is be patient and consistent with the process. The product you are using is not a magic spell, so it requires time and consistency before you begin to see the results.

Generally, aim to use a skincare product for at least six weeks, once or twice daily, to notice a difference. However, remember that sunscreen is only going to protect your skin from further damage. You need to use other products for improvement. For that, you are more than welcome to visit my website www.biotherapyesthetics.com.

Follow these steps in order to take care of your skin other than just using sunscreens.

- The first step is to use a cleanser and a sponge to remove the cleanser from your skin while warm water is forever best.

- The second step is to use the toner (lotion) to finish cleansing the pores.

- The third step is, of course, the glycolic acid, which you will find extremely important to your facial treatment.

- The fourth step is to use a clay mask and silk amino mask. It is one of the best masks available on the market. You will find it at the biotherapy esthetics line.

- Apply the mask on top of the glycolic acid all over your face, neck, and delicate areas. Leave the mask for ten good minutes.

- Remove the mask with a washcloth and warm water.

- Follow up with toner again.

- Applying eye cream, face moisturizer, and sunblock is a must.

- Always remember, it is greatly beneficial to give a facial to yourself during nighttime.

- Apply a good amount of super firming nighttime cream.

- Again, you will find it at the biotherapy skincare line.

The next day, your skin will feel silky soft and youthful. The biotherapy esthetics skincare line is amazingly effective and contains the best ingredients. I am not saying it because it's my product line. I am saying it because I have seen the results myself. You will see the difference in your skin right after using the products.

It took me a very long time to develop this incredible product line for women's and men's skin and beauty. Every single product has been studied and tested in the absolute best ways. Some of the best-sellers are the eye cream, oxygen cleanser, and super firming nighttime cream. They all have amazing results. The best part is that my skincare line is for all skin types. It works more effectively on mature skin. Skincare is my hobby and adds to the beauty as well.

While helping other women with their beauty needs, I feel rewarded at the end of the day. So you can tell how carefully

I would have selected the ingredients and came up with this wonderful product line for you all.

Since this chapter revolves around the sun and how it can affect our skin, let us stick to the subject for now and look at why people resist using sunscreens and a few of many common myths related to it.

Common Myths about Sunscreens

People are often affected by the myths around sunscreens and how they offer skin protection. Learning about them ensures that you develop a better understanding of the underlying science and stay away from myths that may damage your skin. I want to clarify and acknowledge them all because I need you to start taking this one thing seriously for healthy skin. To help people use sunscreen correctly, understanding the truth about them is quite significant. Hence, I am putting it all here for you to learn.

Sunscreen Is Not Always Necessary

Many people believe that sunscreen is necessary only when their entire body is exposed to sunlight. They limit it to specific occasions like going to the pool or when swimming in the ocean. What they do not know is that no matter how much of their skin is exposed to the sun, ultraviolet light is still harmful.

Some people also believe that they do not need to wear sunscreen on cloudy days, which is not true. Just because the sun does not feel as strong as usual does not mean it's not effective. The truth is that even on an overcast day, every time your body is exposed to light from the sun, it is exposed to UV rays.

The common areas that are usually left exposed throughout the day are lower arms and face, which may increase their risk of sun damage. It is best to consider other protective methods like wearing a hat and shades while also covering the exposed skin with sunscreen.

Vitamin D Is Not Absorbed by the Body while Wearing a Sunscreen

The body makes it easily through exposure to UV rays since vitamin D is a vital nutrient for human health. However, sunscreen blocks UV rays. So, in theory, sunscreen prevents a person from getting the proper level of vitamin D by using it 100% of the time.

However, while sunscreen loses its effectiveness over time, sunlight can penetrate clothing. There is also a possibility that a person will forget to put sunscreen on every time they see the sun. Numerous scientists and dermatologists suggest that the proper amount of vitamin D in the body can be created only by five to 30 minutes of sun exposure per day.

Sunscreen Causes Health Problems

This myth originates from an older study done on oxybenzone, one of the active ingredients in many sunscreens. In a lab test, rats exposed to oxybenzone experienced severe adverse side effects. However, researchers used very high levels of exposure in this study to fabricate health problems in the rats.

Their calculation exhibits that these results were unattainable in humans, even those who use sunscreen regularly and liberally. The researchers also noticed that there are no published studies that demonstrate toxic effects in humans caused by absorbed oxybenzone, even after 40 years of its use in sunscreens.

You Do Not Need Sunscreen If You Are Dark-Skinned

People with dark skin are still at risk of sunburn and skin damage. Taking precautions is always recommended, such as wearing sunscreen, regardless of skin color. Some people believe that they do not need to use sunscreen with more melanin in their skin. This is mainly because it protects against sunburns to some extent because it acts to diffuse UVB rays.

Even if people with darker skin are more protected from the sun, they should use a full-spectrum sunscreen. If you also think this way, UVA damage can lead to premature skin aging and wrinkles because it is not blocked by melanin in the same way as sunscreens.

If you plan on spending long hours in the sun unprotected, remember that melanin will not protect your skin from extreme sun exposure. You are at risk of developing skin cancer, even if you have darker skin.

One study shows that skin cancer survival rates are the lowest in people with darker skin, including Asian-Americans, African-Americans, Native Americans, and Pacific Islanders. Hence, these results show that better sunscreen use is equally essential for all skin colors and types, and we surely need to raise awareness of the risk of skin cancer.

Tanning Beds Provide a Protective Base Tan

Some people are made to believe that they should use tanning beds before exposing themselves to a lot of sun rays or to get a quick tan before summer arrives, especially when on vacation. While the sun includes both UVA and UVB light, tanning beds use a high concentration of UVA light to darken the skin quickly. A tanning bed exposes your body to a high level of UVA light, which creates a temporary tan that will not protect the skin much from sun exposure and sunburn caused by UVB light. Therefore, tanning beds should not be considered while opting to protect your skin. They sure have their side effects.

Makeup Is Enough for Face Protection

While there is no doubt that makeup may provide some protection from the sun for a while, it is not enough and indeed not a replacement for a good sunscreen. Makeup should not be seen as the only layer of protection. It should be treated as an additional layer of protection whose primary purpose is aesthetic.

It Is Better to Use Sunscreen Rather than Covering Up

It can be exciting to believe that a layer of sunscreen makes the body invulnerable to the sun. Even if much of their skin is exposed, many people who wear sunscreen believe that it allows them to stay protected throughout the day.

The reality is that if there is anything better than wearing sunscreen, it's covering up the skin. A lot of research studies indicate that covering offers much better protection than sunscreen. Full-coverage clothing with a long-brimmed hat will protect the skin better than any sunscreen.

You Cannot Tan while Wearing Sunscreen

Sunscreen protects the skin from most of the light rays, but some still reach the skin. So, no matter if you are wearing sunscreen, sunlight will still reach your skin. Sunscreen may not entirely protect the body, but it helps protect against most

UVA and UVB rays. Even when someone applies sunscreen multiple times throughout the day, there is still a possibility of getting a tan. The body's natural protective response, when exposed to UV rays, is tanning. Hence, it is best to apply sunscreen and cover up with other things to avoid getting a tan.

All Sunscreens Are the Same

There is a common misconception that all sunscreens are the same and do the same job. However, they may protect against different levels of sun exposure. There are undoubtedly a variety of ingredients present in different sunscreens.

Active ingredients like zinc oxide, titanium dioxide, and ecamsule are often used to filter out UVB and UVA rays. There are also chemical blockers like avobenzone. All the ingredients have their own way of blocking out the sun. Using a full-spectrum sunscreen is crucial because it will protect the skin against the entire range of UV light.

Another crucial thing to consider while buying a sunblock is the sun protection factor (SPF). You must regularly apply sunscreen with an SPF of 15 or higher, even on cloudy days.

This practice is also recommended by the United States Food & Drug Administration (FDA).

Applying Sunscreen Once Lasts All Day

Many people think that sunscreen will last all day after applying it only once. In actual use, sunscreen loses its effectiveness over a short period and breaks down in the light. People should at least apply sunscreen every two to four hours.

Sunscreen Is Waterproof

Sunscreens labeled as sweat-resistant or water-resistant or marketed as sunscreen for sports may appear waterproof. Unfortunately, this is an overstatement of what sunscreen can do. No sunscreen product can be 100% waterproof. People must always reapply water-resistant sunscreen after being exposed to water. Before going into the water, allow the sunscreen to settle on the skin for at least 10 to 15 minutes.

Sunscreen Never Expires

Contrary to popular belief, sunscreen naturally expires. Everything has a shelf life, so does the sunscreen. However, there is often no harm in using an expired sunscreen, yet it may leave the skin unprotected. It occurs since the active ingredients can break down over time, lowering the offered protection.[15]

Toxic and Non-Toxic Ingredients in Sunscreen

Of course, some sunscreens do contain chemical or mineral active ingredients to protect you from the sun. Based on the ingredients, sunscreens can be toxic or non-toxic. The ingredients in the sunscreens should not be irritating, nor should they cause skin allergies. They should be able to withstand the powerful UV radiation without losing effectiveness.

---

[15]https://www.medicalnewstoday.com/articles/318290#Twelve-myths-about-sunscreen

Toxic-Ingredients

Before they can protect us from the radiation of the sun, chemical sunscreens like octinoxate, oxybenzone, avobenzone, and octisalate must be absorbed into the skin. These ingredients absorb the sun rays to protect the skin. They then convert those rays into heat that is released from the skin. But these are also the ingredients of concern. Let's look at each one individually.

Oxybenzone

It is one of the most commonly used sunscreen chemicals. It is linked to organ system toxicity, endocrine disruption, photo allergies, and contact allergies, but exposure to light is required to generate an allergic response. This ingredient, sometimes called benzophenone-3, is often confused with benzophenone, which is another ordinary sunscreen ingredient. Oxybenzone is also harmful to aquatic life, so much that in 2018, Hawaii banned it to protect coral reefs.

It is a commonly used UV filter that does not protect the skin from UVA sun rays but UVB rays. It may be listed as OMC - methoxy-cinnamate or Ethylhexylmethoxy-cinnamate on the packaging. Octinoxate is associated with reproductive toxicity and endocrine disruption by an abundance of data. Researchers have detected this chemical in urine, breast milk, and blood. Since it harms coral reefs, this ingredient was targeted in Hawaii's ban, like oxybenzone.

Homosalate

To prevent direct skin exposure, it is a common sunscreen ingredient that absorbs only UVB rays. This ingredient is associated with hormonal disruption and may intensify the absorption of pesticides, including bug sprays. It may also add to the penetration of other harmful ingredients found within the formulation. This ingredient does not break down readily and is persistent in the environment.

Nanoparticles

Nanoparticles can be a thousand times smaller than the width of a human hair. They are most frequently found as nanoparticle titanium dioxide of zinc oxide. Nanoparticles have not been properly evaluated for their potential effects on environmental health or humans. Researchers are still looking to find its potential effects. But nanoparticles may be more chemically reactive because of their infinitesimally small size. Therefore, they are fast-tracked into the body, meaning they are more bioavailable.

Non-Toxic Ingredients

Like there are some toxic ingredients present in the sunscreens, there are some non-toxic ingredients as well. Let's find out.

Titanium Dioxide

Found in the earth's crust, it is a naturally-occurring mineral. It is a UV absorber, which means it can soak up UV rays. Titanium dioxide may not provide full UVA protection. However, it absorbs UVB rays and some UVA rays. This non-nanoparticle, titanium dioxide, is safe for people and the planet.

Zinc Oxide

Zinc oxide is a naturally-occurring UV absorber. Since zinc oxide protects against both UVA and UVB rays, it offers broad-spectrum protection. Zinc is safe for the environment and humans when in the form of a nanoparticle.[16]

Why Should You Choose Mineral-Based Sunscreen?

As opposed to chemical sunscreen, mineral sunscreen is what precisely it sounds like. A sunscreen that uses minerals, most frequently titanium dioxide and zinc oxide, to safeguard from the sun. The minerals reflect UV rays, so they do not reach you. They sit on the edge of your skin like tiny protective particles. Chemical sunscreens work by absorbing the rays through a chemical reaction. Your body still absorbs the chemicals, and the chemicals can flow into your bloodstream, while this process prevents rays from burning your skin.

Since mineral sunscreen is not absorbed as much as chemical formulas, it's considered the more non-toxic option. Plus point, it's better for the environment. However, just because a sunscreen says it's mineral does not always mean it does not also contain chemicals. Look for options

---

[16]https://www.madesafe.org/education/whats-in-that/sunscreen/

that claim 100% mineral-based active ingredients and research the ingredients of any sunscreen you are unsure about.[17]

---

[17]https://theeverygirl.com/the-best-non-toxic-sunscreens/

Chapter 4- Eating Healthy

They say you are what you eat, but no one takes this statement seriously. When in actuality, eating well is crucial to good health and physical well-being. Eating healthy helps us maintain a healthy weight and reduces our risk of high blood pressure, type-2 diabetes, high cholesterol, and the risk of developing cardiovascular disease and even cancers. It's better to be safe than sorry, so why take risks, especially when it comes to your physical health?

Other than healthier skin, eating healthy has many other benefits to offer. Have you ever noticed that we have more energy, better concentration, and better sleep when we begin to eat healthily? All of these ingredients add up to happier and healthier lives. So what makes you think that eating healthy is not important?

The more you make it easy for yourself, the more you will be interested in keeping up with this huge lifestyle change. Healthy eating, for everyone, should be an enjoyable social experience. When people eat and drink healthy, they get all the essential nutrients they need for proper development and growth while maintaining a good relationship with food and their environment.

As an aesthetician, my responsibility is to help guide you to build a life where you have not only healthy skin but also a healthy body since they both are interlinked. I have five important rules that I live by. Let me put them out for you.

5 Rules to Follow

It is not easy for a lot of people to follow a healthy lifestyle. Especially if you are someone with a busy schedule trapped inside a lazy body, it might seem incredibly complicated. Whereas advertisements and experts all around you seem to give conflicting advice. Nothing about leading a healthy life is complicated, nor is it something impossible for you to follow. Remember, you need to lose weight to gain optimal health and feel better every day. Hence, all you need to do is follow these five simple rules.

Rule No. 1: Do Not Put Toxins into Your Body

Numerous studies show what all people put in their bodies is downright toxic for their health. As I talked in my chapters earlier, some toxins such as cigarettes, alcohol, and abusive drugs, which are also highly addictive, make it hard for people to avoid them or give them up completely.

Diet and exercise should be your least concern if you have a problem with one of these substances. Of course, this doesn't mean that you should completely discard them. Tobacco and other abusive drugs are bad for everyone, while alcohol is fine in moderation for those who can tolerate it. I need you to take this first rule seriously and stay firm on your decision, not to put toxins into your body.

Rule No. 2: Avoid Junk Food

Eating unhealthy is an even more common problem today, with all these new restaurants and food ventures coming in. The root cause is the constant promotion of junk foods. Believe me; you need to minimize the consumption of these unhealthy foods if you really want to gain optimal health. Cutting down on the consumption of processed and packaged foods is undoubtedly the single most effective change needed to improve your diet.

It can be tough because many of these foods are designed to be extremely tasty and extremely hard to resist. But when you keep an ideal image of yourself as your ultimate goal, nothing can stop you. Look for ingredients. Added sugars are among the worst when it comes to specific ingredients. These include sucrose and high-fructose corn syrup.

It is also a good idea to avoid all trans fats, which are found in some types of margarine and packaged baked foods. At the end of the day, your goal is to avoid junk foods.

Rule No. 3: Nourish Your Body with Real Foods

The simple and most effective way to have a healthy diet is to focus on nature. It's about maintaining a balance by consuming a combination of animals and plants - fish, meat, eggs, vegetables, fruits, seeds, almonds, walnuts, as well as healthy fats, oils, and high-fat dairy products.

If you are healthy, lean, and active, then eating whole, unrefined carbs is absolutely fine. These include potatoes, legumes, and whole grains such as oats. Sources lead to dramatic improvements. People subconsciously start eating less simply by cutting back on carbohydrates, which can help lose a lot of weight.

You will have to make an effort to choose whole, unprocessed foods in whatever you do, instead of foods that look like they are made in a factory. Choosing whole, unprocessed foods such as vegetables, fruits, whole grains, and seeds is particularly important for your health. This is what I mean when I say that nourish your body with real foods.

Rule No. 4: You Need to Stick with It for Life

You need to change your perspective as a whole and look at processed food as your health's greatest enemy. During the COVID-19 pandemic, a lot of different food companies started offering food deliveries for lunch and dinner. It is the easiest way to get these services delivered to our dinner table during our difficult times in the country worldwide. But as I was looking at what the food possesses, I chose not to eat it.

Remember, a dieting mindset is bad because it almost never works in the long term. You might be wondering why it is critical to bring about a change in your lifestyle for this one particular reason. Being healthy is not a sprint but a marathon. It will be best if you stick to it for life because it takes a whole lot of time to build such habits. It is that one change needed to stay healthy in life.

Rule No. 5: Education and Wellness

You need to be educated about all the ingredients and know the difference between unhealthy and healthy food. At the same time, your brain requires attention. Brainpower is important. You need to go out of your way to take care of it. As we talk about education and wellness, here are a few tips for you to follow.

- Eat a variety of healthy foods.

- Base your diet on plenty of foods that are not rich in carbohydrates.

- Replace saturated with unsaturated fat.

- Enjoy plenty of fruits and vegetables.

- Reduce salt and sugar intake.

- Eat regularly and control the portion size.

- Drink plenty of fluids.

- Maintain healthy body weight.

How Do You Use the Right Products?

What kind of daily routine do you need to follow? There can be many such questions emerging in your brain. Just relax. I am here to answer them all. I will find the easiest ways to explain to you what products are right for your skin and how you should use them.

If you have been following my book well, you must already know that skin is the body's largest organ. Our face and body need to be treated with the right products, and we all must follow a very proper skincare routine.

Let's go back to where we discussed the layers of our skin. Our skin is divided into a lot of different layers. The first three layers are the most important and need to be taken care of in special ways with the right products.

The first layer is what we call the epidermis. The second layer is called the dermis, whereas germinative is the deepest epidermal layer. The germinative layer attaches the epidermis to the basal lamina, below which lies the layers of the dermis. Let's look at some facts.

Do you know where the thinnest skin of your body is located? It's that of your eyelids. Contrarily, the thickest skin is on the palms and soles of the feet. As time passes and we look at our skin, we wonder: how many skin types are there? Well, to give an overview, normally there are three skin types: dry, oily, and a combination of the two. Not sure how to keep each type healthy? Don't worry. I have it covered.

Good skin is not just a matter of DNA, as not everyone is lucky enough to be born with perfect skin. You have to take care of your daily habits, keeping track of what you feed your body, both internally and externally. We do not often realize this, but our habits greatly impact what we see in the mirror.

Depending on what product reviews you read or doctors you consult, there are numerous abrupt opinions on everything, from moisturizing your skin to protecting it from the ultraviolet rays. Here are a few things you should keep in mind to sort through all the noise. *Always remember that it is never too late to start.*

Your skincare routine should consist of the three following steps.

1. Cleansing: Washes your face

2. Toning: Balances the skin

3. Moisturizing: Hydrates and softens the skin

The final goal of any skincare routine is to tune your skin complexion so that it's functioning at its best. Another important goal is to troubleshoot or diagnose any areas you need to work on. However, being an aesthetician, I have come up with a skincare routine that I believe everyone must follow. This is going to help you heal your skin and be confident about yourself as you head out of your house.

Skincare Routine

Follow up on your diet plan with a proper skincare routine. Remember that you need to cover all the things that are related to your skin. Our eventual goal is to look and feel young. Therefore, take care of all the aspects related to your skin. Here are the steps you must follow along with a healthy diet plan.

Step 1: Base Cleanser

How do you use a cleanser? Some oil-based cleansers are designed to spell a cast on wet skin, while others are best on dry skin. Always read the instructions before applying a small amount to your skin. You need to massage and rinse with water before drying with a clean towel.

The right products are very effective and shall lead to wonderful results. They must feel safe on your epidermis. I highly recommend the Biotherapy Esthetics Skincare product line. The cleanser has oxygen in it. It leaves the pores cleaned and gives them enough space to breathe.

Finding Your Facial Cleanser

The right formula to keep your skin healthy is plundering essential healthy oils. Take it easy with exfoliating scrubs, use them once a week, and avoid those with crushed walnut shells or abrasive ingredients. So when choosing the right cleanser for your skin, here's what to look for. The best for all skin types is the oxygenate cleanser with oxygen in it to open up the pores of your skin and be able to remove all the impurities from your epidermis.

Step 2: Toner or Lotion (They Have The Same Functionality but Different Names)

What are toners? Toners are designed to remove dead cells and dirt left behind after cleansing while replenishing skin through hydration. How do you use it? You either need to tap onto the skin or a cotton pad straight after cleansing directly. Swipe it over the face in an outward motion for better results. I highly recommend toners to all my clients and now readers. We often don't realize it, but they are very much needed for the skin. Also, some toners have the ability to minimize the pores, hence creating a protective shield.

How to Use a Toner

For a lot of people, the word *toner* brings to mind stinging astringent from the '80s. The earliest was an alcohol-based product that was used to dry up oily skin and remove all the leftover dirt following the cleansing. Dr. Nazarian says that today's formulas, however, have evolved. Think of them as supplements. These thin liquids give out an extra shot of nutrients, absorbing other products in your regimen better, penetrating the third layer of the skin while still balancing your complexion.

Most experts, including an esthetician from New York City, Jordana Mattioli, say that consider toner to be optional. It can be a great way to add another layer of skin-replenishment. Here are some best ingredients to look for if you have the time and inclination.

-     Alpha and Hyaluronic acid to boost hydration, seal in dewiness, and plump skin to subtly treat fine lines

- Moreover, vitamins E and C to fight daily exposure to free radicals that can age your skin

Remember that the toner is very important and you must look for the right ingredients. Again, Biotherapy Esthetics has the toner with the best and secure ingredients the skin needs. They help protect your skin in the best possible way. Always check whether the product is comedogenic or not.

What Does Non-Comedogenic Mean Exactly?

This term frequency appears on product labels, and we often hear it from the skincare experts. However, it is not always defined in simple, clear language. Here is a quick explanation. If a product claims to be non-comedogenic, it means it should not clog your pores or trigger acne either by occluding the skin, blocking glands, or irritating the hair follicle.

A number of companies do their internal tests to determine whether a product should be contemplated comedogenic or not. However, the claim is not regulated by the FDA. Some usually known comedogenic ingredients are cocoa butter and coconut oil. Typically, the lesser the ingredients a product has, the easier it is to determine if it will cause any reaction or not.

Step 3: Anti-oxidants Serum

You may wonder what these serums are and why you need them. I am here to clarify that for you. A serum based on anti-oxidants will protect your skin from unstable molecules. Since serums have a high concentration of certain ingredients, all you need is the anti-oxidant one. Vitamins C and E are common anti-oxidants used to improve the firmness and texture of the skin. Others to look out for include resveratrol, green tea, and caffeine.

How to Use Serum

To use it, just put a few drops onto your face and neck. A bottle to try is Biotherapy Esthetics EC Ferulic. It promises to protect against UVA and UVB rays while diminishing aging signs. For a more affordable alternative, try Botanical Bio Peptide concentrate serum. You will also find it at the Biotherapy Aesthetics.

Why Use Serum?

The serum is yet another helpful product that is needed by our skin. Simply put, serums are powerful skin allies. These elixirs can surely counter a number of issues, since they are filled with concentrated doses of active ingredients, from wrinkles to dark spots. Even if you don't have any particular issues, from dark spots to wrinkles, we all need a common antioxidant serum in the morning to safeguard our skin from daily attackers. While there are countless options for ingredients to handle any such issues, look for these products.

Hyaluronic Acid: To seal in hydration and strengthen the barrier function (the top layer of your skin) to prevent moisture loss.

Vitamin C: To help brighten dull skin and decrease dark spots with continued use

Retinol, Vitamin B3, and Peptide: To restore elastin and collagen production, proteins in the body that help shut outlines and skin sagging.

Do not try mixing a serum into your moisturizer to save time. This decreases the ability of the serum to absorb effectively. Dr. Nazarian says that she prefers antioxidants in the morning because they give you additional protection from the environment, and most of us do not use enough sunscreen. Yet certain ingredients react best when slathered at night. Take the example of retinol. They are not sun-stable and will degrade if applied in the daytime.

Step 4: Eye Cream

Eye cream is an entirely new concept for some people. However, they do not know that the skin around the eyes tends to be thinner and more sensitive. It is also prone to signs of aging, including puffiness, fine lines, and darkness. A good eye cream will not completely eliminate all your issues. However, it can brighten, smooth, and firm up the area.

How to Use Eye Cream

Just dab a small amount using your ring finger onto the eye area. Don't forget to be gentle.

Why Use Eye Cream?

Can you survive without an eye cream? Trust me; you cannot. You really need an eye cream because the skin around the eyes is quite thin, delicate, and more likely to react to irritation than other areas.

Caffeine, peptides, and hyaluronic acid are also found to be soothing for under-eye bags and inflammation. However, dark circles can be visible in veins or actual discoloration common in darker skin tones. They need to be taken care of. When buying an eye cream, look for brightening ingredients like vitamin C, kojic acid, and niacinamide.

Step 5: Lighter Face Oil or Any Kind of Serum

Lighter products should be applied earlier as they are easily absorbable. So the next time you apply a moisturizer, remember that light face oil needs to be applied first. They are especially useful if your skin is showing signs of flakiness, dehydration, or dryness.

How to Use It

After squeezing a few drops onto your fingertips, gently rub them to warm the oil. Once you think it's warm enough, lightly dab onto your face.

Step 6: Moisturizer

What is a moisturizer? A moisturizer smooths and softens your skin and hence is mandatory. People with dry skin type must opt for a cream or balm. In this case, thicker creams provide you with the best solution. They work best on normal or combination skin, which is why fluids are recommended for oilier skin types. Effective products include glycerin, ceramides, antioxidants, and peptides.

How to Use It

- Take a good amount on your palm.

- Apply on to your skin.

- Massage it until it is completely absorbed in your skin.

- Always use upward strokes.

Why Use Moisturizer?

Moisturizers are used for the primary function of keeping your skin soft and hydrated. Moisturizers form a protective layer over your skin that minimizes water loss, according to Dr. Charles. They can also complement the naturally found protective oils as well as other building blocks within the skin, such as ceramides. These are the products that doctors recommend using all year round for all skin types. Our skin naturally loses the ability to retain moisture as we age, which is why I highly recommend using moisturizers daily. Frequent washing can strip natural hydrating agents from the surface, which makes it an even more important ingredient of your skincare routine.

Step 7: Night Cream

Night cream focuses on repairing the damage done to your skin during the day with thicker products at night. At this time, use anything that makes your skin sensitive to sunlight, including physical exfoliates and chemical peels. They serve as the best therapists for your skin after a long and tiring day.

Morning creams have certain ingredients in them that act as a shield for your skin from environmental aggressors that you may come in contact with. Many contain antioxidants with a light-weight consistency to minimize pollution-based free radicals and sunscreen to shield you from ultraviolet radiation.

On the other hand, night creams focus on repairing any damage you may have suffered with ingredients like retinol to speed cellular turnover and counteract dark spots. These creams also replenish moisture levels with emollients that often create a rich, thick texture.

Step 8: Hydrating Mask

Masks are best in clay, designed to clean the skin's pores and deliver long-lasting moisture.

How to Use a Clay Mask

Apply an oxygen cleanser, then apply a thin layer of glycolic acid to the skin. Apply the mask right after that to your face and neck. Leave the mask on for 10 minutes, then remove it with warm water using a sponge or washcloth. Sea sponges are the best for all skin types.

Why Use Masks?

Are face masks actually worth all the buzz around them? To say that face masks have become popular lately is a bit of an understatement. According to Dr. Nazarian from NYC, masks offer highly concentrated treatment to address specific issues. Clay masks are actually the best for oily skin type. Let's look at its functionality.

Clay Masks

These masks absorb oil and can have a mild exfoliating effect; hence, they are great for oily skin areas. Leave the clay mask on for 10 minutes and wash it off with warm water. Apply clay mask right after serum but before the moisturizer.

Note that masks should be used in moderation. Not more than once a week to prevent any sort of irritation or reaction.

Now that you know the skincare routine, you need to follow one golden rule.

Give It Time

Everything in life takes time, patience, and persistence, and so does your skin to heal. Our skin goes through a lot every day, which often goes unnoticed by us being human beings. It is why I stress so much about taking care of your skin and having a healthy skincare routine. However, as you try to follow up on a healthy diet plan and a balanced skincare routine, remember that there is no magic spell to healthy skin. It will take time for sure.

According to Dr. Rachel Nazarian, who is a Manhattan dermatologist at SchweigerDermotogu group, the science behind skincare products has been studied quite comprehensively and has progressed over time. However, there is no such thing as an immediate fix. You need time to reap the benefits. Results can only be seen through consistent use of the products that are a part of your skincare routine. As I said earlier, try to use a product once or twice every day for at least six weeks before you can notice a difference.

Pro tip: Stay consistent with the quantity of any skincare product that you apply, from thinnest to thickest layer. For instance, cleanser, toner, serum if you use it, and then moisturizer.

Our Skin Goes through a Lot

According to the New York City Dermatologist, Dr. Carlos Charles, washing your face is one of the most basic yet indispensable steps of any routine. Our skin comes in contact with numerous environmental pollutants, dirt, and other factors every day that should be gently removed. Wash your face twice a day. Start and end your day by washing it to avoid clogged pores, dullness, and acne.

Back to the eating habits, let's look at a few natural ingredients that can help keep our skin healthy, but first, let's talk about collagen.

What Is Collagen?

Collagen is the most familiar protein found in the body. It's present in tendons, fat, and ligaments, among other places. It is crucial to our bone structure's strength. When collagen level is healthy, our cells that contain collagen take on a strong and youthful appearance.

Elastin is another kind of protein present in the body. It is found in places of our body that contract, such as arteries and lungs. This happens because of elastin's one outstanding characteristic: the ability to snap back into place and maintain its original shape.

Elastin and collagen are both proteins that can be found in your skin. They work together to give skin its shape and texture. Skin with a healthy level of both collagen and elastin is not only more youthful but also stronger. Interestingly, stimulating the growth of collagen causes a domino effect. This means the more collagen you have, the better your body will produce and maintain itself.

Ways to Boost Collagen

One study suggests that hyaluronic acid can help boost collagen production in the human body. Hyaluronic is a naturally found acid in the body, but it decreases as we age. Eating foods rich in amino acids and vitamin C can increase the hyaluronic acid level and collagen in the body. They both are important for the skin. The foods rich in vitamin C Ginseng, Cilantro, and Algae can also help boost collagen. The easiest way to boost collagen in your body is by using collagen peptides. Simply look for products that have peptides in them.

Now let's look at the ingredients present in nature that can be really healthy for your skin.

Aloe Vera

Aloe vera is simply the potato of all the natural remedies related to physical health. Just like potato goes with every vegetable, aloe vera gel goes with everything you mix it with. You can mix it with cream and apply it overnight for great skin. You can mix it with hair oil in case you are facing hair problems or when you have to deal with after-wax rashes. You can even apply aloe vera gel if you get a sunburn. You can apply it after threading as well to help the skin heal and avoid redness.

Aloe vera produces two healing substances used for medicine. The gel is obtained from the cells in the center of the leaf. The latex is obtained from the cells just beneath the leaf skin. It contains minerals, anti-oxidant vitamins, and eight different enzymes. If you ever get the time, just read about this one plant, and you will be amazed by the benefits it hides.

Fresh aloe vera gel is traditionally used in India as a medicine for constipation, worm infestation, and as a natural remedy for colic (severe pain in the abdomen caused by several reasons). It is most commonly used as a remedy for skin problems like burns, sunburns, frostbite, itches, cold sores, and psoriasis (a skin condition that speeds the life cycle of skin cells resulting in painful patches).

Aloe vera gel has long been used for healing and soothing wounds. It works to treat cuts and burns because the aloe vera plant increases collagen production when applied topically or taken orally. This cell growth-stimulating property can help boost collagen production in your skin. Aloe vera can be applied directly to the skin in pure form or in the many products available on the market containing aloe vera.

I personally suggest applying one of the vital hydrant toner (aloe vera gel) from Biotherapy Esthetics products, which consists of more than 80% aloe vera gel. It helps firm your skin. You will notice the difference in your skin within the first four weeks. Always use it after cleansing the skin with a strong cleanser and after applying the vital hydrant toner gel.

Lean it on, and following up with night-time cream, super firming cream, eye cream always is super important, not only on the area around your eyes but also the area between brows and upper lip area.

What Not to Do

If you are trying to help your skin look younger and healthier, make sure you are not burning your skin in the sun or the tanning bed. Smoking can also damage your skin prematurely, so avoid it as much as you can. One way of maintaining a healthy glow is by spending time outside with the sunscreen's protection, but trying to avoid the things that you know are harmful to your skin is another best way to protect your skin.

Some collagen supplements do have side effects. The most common ones are allergic reactions, calcium overproduction, and joint pain. If you have an allergic reaction to seafood or meat products, be very careful when taking any kind of collagen supplement. The next thing you may ask is:

How Can I Keep My Skin Thick as I Age?

Well, a lot of it has to do with what you put inside your body. You must take care of your diet. Fruits and vegetables, along with whole grains, proteins, and vitamin E, must be included in your diet. Keep looking for foods rich in minerals and protein. They can mainly be found in foods such as almonds and avocados. They can also support skin health. The fats in these foods may help keep the skin healthy and thick, which is good to keep you look younger than your age.

The skin is the fastest and largest growing organ of the human body. However, for some people, it can grow too fast, caused by a condition called scleroderma. Although the cause of the disease is unknown, experts say it results in an overproduction of collagen in the body. Having thick skin is not always a good thing. Drinking enough water helps to keep the skin hydrated.

At this point, you may wonder, what are some other benefits of eating healthy?

Benefits of Eating Healthy

A well-balanced diet will give you all the energy you may need throughout the day. It keeps you active and provides you with nutrients you may need for growth and repair. It helps you stay healthy and physically strong, at the same time, preventing you from diseases related to diet, for instance, different types of cancers.

Moreover, the best part about eating healthy is that it helps you maintain a healthy weight. It also helps you maintain some of the essential vitamins and minerals needed by your body.

Let's look at some major diseases that you can prevent yourself from by opting for a healthy lifestyle.

Reduced Cancer Risks

An unhealthy diet leads to obesity, which may increase a person's risk of developing cancer. A healthy weight helps reduce the risk of many diseases, including lethal cancers. Diets rich in fruits and vegetables actually prevent you from chronic diseases.

Many phytochemicals found in vegetables, fruits, legumes, and nuts act as antioxidants, which protect cells from damage that can cause cancer. Some of these antioxidants include lycopene, beta-carotene, and vitamins A, C, and E.

Type-2 Diabetes

Along with a healthy weight and a balanced diet that's low in saturated fat and high in fiber found in whole grains can help to reduce your risk of developing type-2 diabetes. Isn't that amazing?

Heart Health

By maintaining cholesterol level and blood pressure, a healthy diet rich in vegetables, fruits, low-fat dairy, and whole grains can help to reduce your risk of heart disease. If you experience high blood pressure and cholesterol symptoms, you need to check that you may be consuming too much salt and saturated fats in your diet.

Blood clots can often lead to heart attacks. There is some evidence that vitamin E may prevent blood clots from forming. The following foods contain high levels of vitamin E.

- Peanuts

- Almonds

- Hazelnuts

- Green vegetables

- Sunflower seed

Medical professionals have long recognized the link between trans fats and heart-related illnesses such as coronary heart disease. It will help reduce their low-density lipoprotein cholesterol level when a person eliminates trans fats from the diet. This type of cholesterol causes plaque to gather within the arteries, increasing stroke risk and the risk of a heart attack.

Limiting the consumption of salt to 1,500 milligrams a day can help reduce blood pressure levels, which is also essential for heart health. Many processed and fast foods contain salt. A person hoping to lower their blood pressure should avoid these.

Strong Bones and Teeth

Having strong bones has a lot to do with looking young, so as much as your skin is important, you must never neglect the role bones play in keeping you young and active. A diet abundant in calcium keeps your teeth and bones strong and can help to slow down bone loss (osteoporosis) associated with getting older.

Usually, calcium is associated with dairy products, but you can also get calcium by eating dark green vegetables such as broccoli, kale, pilchards, tinned salmon (with bones) or sardines, or calcium-fortified foods such as fruit juices, cereals, and soy products.

How to Manage Your Weight?

Maintaining a healthy diet that includes lots of vegetables, fruit, whole grains, and a moderate amount of unsaturated fats, dairy, and meat can help you maintain a steady and healthy weight. When you make a good variety of these foods a part of your daily eating, it leaves smaller room for high sugar and fat foods - a leading cause of weight gain.

Eating a healthy diet in the right amount along with a healthy amount of exercise can also help you lose weight, maintain healthy blood pressure, lower cholesterol levels, and decrease your risk of type-2 diabetes. All in all, if you intend to control your weight and stay healthy, you will have to put in the time and effort required to do so.

Chapter 5- Exercising

How do you define exercise? It is defined as an essential movement that burns calories in your body and makes your muscles work better. There are numerous types of exercises that you can involve yourself in, including walking, running, swimming, dancing, and jogging. However, a lot of people do not understand how important it is to exercise.

When you are physically active, it benefits your health in a number of ways, both physically and mentally. It may even help you live a healthier and longer life. We have all heard that various medical practitioners emphasize the importance of exercise, but have you ever wondered why they are so adamant about it? Let's look at a few reasons that shed light on the importance of exercise.

Exercise Helps Lose Weight

The first and foremost benefit of exercising is, it helps you lose weight. A lot of people exercise only with this sole purpose even though it has numerous other benefits too. Exercise can help you maintain weight loss and prevent excessive weight gain. You burn calories when you engage yourself in any sort of physical activity. The more intense the activity, the more calories you burn.

Numerous studies show that inactivity is one of the major reasons behind weight gain, which leads to obesity. In order to understand the relationship between exercise and weight reduction, it is important to understand the relationship between energy expenditure and exercise.

Your body puts out the stored energy in three ways: digesting food, maintaining body functions like your heartbeat and breathing, and exercising. A reduced calorie intake while dieting will lower your metabolic rate, which in turn will delay weight loss. Contrarily, it has been observed that regular exercise can increase your metabolic rate, which will help you lose more weight since it burns more calories.

Moreover, studies have shown that combining aerobic exercise with resistance training can speed up fat loss and muscle mass maintenance, which is crucial for maintaining a healthy body. Therefore, exercise is critical to supporting fast metabolism and burning more calories every day.

Visiting the gym on a regular basis is great, but you do not have to worry if you cannot afford to dedicate a huge chunk of your time to exercise every day. Even a small amount of activity is way better than doing nothing at all. You need to get more active throughout the day to reap the true benefits of exercise. Even the slightest changes in your routine can make a difference. For instance, you can rev up your household chores or take the stairs instead of the elevator. However, remember that consistency is the key.

Exercise Helps Maintain Strong Bones and Muscles

Exercise plays a crucial role in maintaining and building strong muscles and bones. Physical activities like weightlifting can encourage muscle building, especially when paired with a sufficient intake of proteins. The reason behind this is that exercise helps release hormones that promote the capability of your muscles to absorb amino acid. This does not only help them grow but also reduces their breakdown.

People tend to lose muscle mass and function as they age, which can lead to disabilities and injuries. A regular physical activity practice is necessary to reduce muscle loss and maintain strength. Moreover, when you are younger, exercise helps build bone density in addition to preventing osteoporosis later in life.

Interestingly, high-impact exercises such as running, gymnastics, or odd-impact sports such as basketball and soccer have appeared to promote a higher bone density than non-impact sports like cycling and swimming. Regardless of the kind, physical activity helps you build muscles and strong bones, hence aiding in osteoporosis prevention.

Exercise Eliminates the Risk of Numerous Diseases

Are you worried about heart diseases? Are you hoping to prevent yourself from developing any heart disease? Then exercise is all you need. Being active boosts high-density lipoprotein (HDL) cholesterol, the good cholesterol, and decreases unhealthy triglycerides from the body. This boost keeps your blood flow smooth, which automatically decreases your risk of cardiovascular diseases.

Just to motivate you enough, let's look at the diseases that can be prevented or managed through exercise.

- Metabolic syndrome

- Stroke

- Type-2 diabetes

- High blood pressure

- Depression

- Anxiety

- Arthritis

- Falls

- Numerous types of cancer

It can also help enhance cognitive function and lessen the risk of death from all chronic medical diseases.[18]

Exercise Improves Mood

If you lack an emotionally stable life or need to blow off steam after a long stressful day, a brisk walk or a gym session can help. Physical activity stimulates a number of brain chemicals that may leave you feeling less anxious, more relaxed, and happier. You may also feel better about yourself and your appearance if you exercise daily, which can upgrade your self-esteem and boost your confidence.

---

[18] Exercise: 7 benefits of regular physical activity
https://www.mayoclinic.org/healthy-lifestyle/fitness/in-depth/exercise/art-20048389

Exercise Boosts Energy

Are you tired of your everyday routine? Perhaps you are a job holder, an entrepreneur, or a housewife who has just got done with the house chores and grocery shopping, feeling tiredness in your bones. Regular physical activity can boost your endurance and improve your muscle strength. Exercise distributes oxygen and nutrients to your tissues and causes your cardiovascular system to work more systematically. You have more energy to tackle day-to-day chores when your heart and lung health is in an improved state.

According to a study, six weeks of regular exercise reduced fatigue level for 36 healthy people who had reported constant fatigue. Other than that, exercise can notably increase energy level for people who have chronic fatigue syndrome (CFS) and other serious diseases.

In reality, exercise appears to be more potent at battling CFS than other treatments, including passive therapies like stretching and relaxation, or no treatment at all. Moreover, exercise has been proven to increase people's energy level suffering from progressive illnesses such as cancer, HIV/AIDS, and multiple sclerosis.

Exercise Can Make You Feel Happier

It has been proven that exercise enhances your mood and decreases feelings of stress, anxiety, and depression. It develops changes in the parts of the brain that regulate anxiety and stress. It can also multiply brain sensitivity for the hormone's serotine and norepinephrine, which alleviate feelings of depression.

Moreover, exercise can grow the production of endorphins, which are known to help reduce the perception of pain and construct positive feelings. Additionally, exercise has been shown to decrease symptoms in people suffering from anxiety. It can also help them practice distraction from their fears and be more aware of their mental state.

Interestingly, it does not matter how extreme your workout is. It appears that your mood can benefit from exercise, no matter the intensity of physical activity. In fact, a study consisting of 24 women who had been diagnosed with depression revealed that exercise of any intensity remarkably reduced feelings of depression.

Exercise affects your mood so strongly that choosing to exercise even makes a difference over short periods. Another study took 26 healthy people as their sample who normally exercised every day. Some of them were asked to continue exercising, while others were stopped for two weeks. Now, the ones who stopped exercising were found to have an increase in their negative energy. Exercising on a regular basis can improve your mood and reduce feelings of anxiety and depression.[19]

Exercise Promotes Better Sleep

Do you have trouble falling asleep? Regular physical activity can help you relax and fall asleep faster, better, and deeper. The energy depletion that takes place during exercise triggers recuperative processes during sleep. Furthermore, the increase in body temperature during exercise is thought to improve sleep quality by dropping during sleep.

According to research, 150 minutes of moderate-to-vigorous activity every week can provide up to 65% improvement in sleep quality. Another research showed that 16 weeks of physical activity improved sleep quality and

---

[19]The Top 10 Benefits of Regular Exercise
https://www.healthline.com/nutrition/10-benefits-of-exercise#TOC_TITLE_HDR_2

helped a number of people with insomnia. They were found to sleep more deeply and longer than the control group. It also helped them feel more energized throughout the day. It also appears to be beneficial for the elderly, especially those who tend to be affected by sleep disorders and must engage in regular exercise.

You can be adaptable to the type of exercise you choose. It appears that either aerobic exercise combined with resistance training or aerobic exercise alone can improve sleep quality. The important tip to remember is, do not exercise too close to the time you go to bed. It can leave you too energized to fall asleep.

Exercise Can Lessen Pain

Chronic pain can be weakening, but exercise can help decrease it. For many years, in fact, the direction for treating chronic pain was inactivity and rest. Nevertheless, a number of recent researches depict that exercise helps with relieving chronic pain.

An overview of numerous studies suggests that exercise helps people with chronic pain and improves their quality of life. Moreover, several studies show that exercise can help control pain that's associated with various health conditions, including fibromyalgia, chronic low back pain, and chronic soft tissue shoulder disorder, to name a few. Other than that, physical activity can also increase pain tolerance and decrease pain perception.[20]

Exercise Helps Improve Your Skin

If I say that exercise is an anti-aging agent, it isn't a false statement. The effects of exercise on the skin are well known. For example, one study found that when your heart beats faster, muscles pump out more of a certain protein, which in turn powers skin cells to act younger. In fact, over time, exercise can make your skin about 25 years younger, at the microscopic level, though. You may not be able to see it physically, but internally, it does the job. It can also help prevent age-related muscle loss, keep your bones strong, improve balance, and, most importantly, reduce the health risk significantly for people aged 65 and over.

Exercise attenuates the major hallmarks of aging. Regular exercise has multi-system anti-aging effects. Let's look at

---

[20]The Top 10 Benefits of Regular Exercise
https://www.healthline.com/nutrition/10-benefits-of-exercise#TOC_TITLE_HDR_11

how exercise impacts the major hallmarks of aging. Your skin can get affected by the amount of oxidative stress that occurs in your body. It occurs when the body's antioxidant defenses cannot entirely mend the damage that is caused by free radicals to the cells. This can deteriorate your skin and damage their internal structures.

Although exhaustive and extreme physical activity can contribute to oxidative harm, regular moderate exercise can escalate the production of natural antioxidants in your body, which help protect cells. In the same way, exercise can trigger blood flow and induce skin cell adaptations that can help delay the appearance of skin aging.

I personally believe that besides searching for normal pharmaceutical targets of the aging cycle, more research efforts should be allocated to gain insight into the molecular medications of the benefits of exercise and to implement effective exercise interventions for older adults.

Exercise and physical activity on cardiovascular risk restrictive studies strongly suggest that regular physical activity is associated with a lower risk of cardiovascular mortality. Recent technological advances have fundamentally altered humans' vocational and lifestyle behaviors in the space of a few generations. They are profound changes associated with exposure to television devices, and the internet has rapidly accelerated an underlying trend in sedentary behavior related to urbanization. So the next time you have a stressful day, remember, exercise is there to relax your body and mind. You know what to do next.

A Few More Benefits of Exercising

We have already talked about the major reasons why it is so important to exercise for your health. However, it is alarming that teens only get 60 minutes or more of moderate-to-vigorous physical activity every day, according to experts. Still, here are some more benefits of the exercise.

- Exercise is beneficial for each part of the body, including the mind.

- Exercise causes the body to produce chemicals that can help a person feel good.

- Exercise can provide people with a real sense of accomplishment and pride at having achieved a goal, like beating the target weight you had set for yourself.

- Exercise helps people maintain a healthy weight.

- Regular exercise lowers a person's risk of developing a number of diseases, including obesity, type-2 diabetes, and high blood pressure.

- Exercise can help a person age well. Your body will surely thank you later, while exercise may not seem important to you right now.

A Few Exercise That You Can Perform

Exercise three times every week, at least. It can bring numerous benefits. Here are a few exercises that you can easily perform at home or outdoors.

Yoga

There are many different ways that you can adopt in your routine to meet your physical needs. Yoga is one of the best exercises you can do at home. Before any routine, of course, you can talk to your healthcare provider. If you are ready to get started with this routine, that is great! But remember to consult your provider first, especially if you have an extensive medical history. Exercise sure is important, but your personal health and safety should always come first.

Aerobic Exercise

Just like every other muscle in our body, the heart enjoys a great workout. Aerobic exercise is a kind of exercise that gets you breathing harder and, in turn, pumps the heart. Your heart, lungs, and other parts of the body get better and stronger at getting oxygen in the form of oxygen-carrying blood cells when you work out regularly.

If you are a sportsperson, you will probably get at least an hour or more of moderate-to-vigorous activity on practice days. A number of sports give you a great aerobic workout, including soccer, basketball, lacrosse, rowing, and hockey. However, you don't have to worry if you are not a sportsperson. There are a number of ways to get the aerobic exercise done. These include running, biking, hiking, swimming, in-line skating, dancing, tennis, walking quickly, and cross-country skiing.

Strength Training

Your heart is not the only muscle that benefits from exercising every day. But other muscles in your body also benefit from the exercise. Your muscles become stronger as you use them while exercising. Strong muscles also play an important role in supporting your physical health because they help stop injuries and strengthen your joints. Building your muscles also help you maintain a healthy weight and burn more calories since muscles also use more energy than fat does.

A healthier way to build muscles is to lift weights. Strength training can also help improve balance and health. Strength training reduces the risk of complications from various chronic health issues like arthritis, diabetes, and osteoporosis.

You don't always have to lift weights to make your bones and muscles stronger. Multiple kinds of exercises strengthen different muscle groups. For instance, try rowing or cross-country skiing for your arms muscles. Those old gym class standbys, I am talking about pull-ups and push-ups, are also great for building arm muscles.

Try running, rowing, skating, or biking for strong legs. Squats and leg raise also work for legs. You can never beat rowing, pilates or yoga, crunches, and planks for abdominal and core strength.

If you are going to try strength training, the crucial thing to remember is that it is not about how quickly you can move or how heavy you can lift, but your body's flexibility is the healthiest improvement. It is what prevents the back, arms, legs, and muscles from aching.

Flexibility Training

Making your heart and other muscles stronger is not the only important goal of exercising. It can also help the body stay flexible, meaning that your muscles and joints stretch and bend easily. When your body is flexible, it may also help improve your performance in sports if you are a sportsperson. Numerous activities, like martial arts or dance, require great flexibility. However, increased flexibility can also help people perform better at other sports such as soccer or lacrosse.

Sports and other activities that uplift flexibility are easy to find. Martial arts like gymnastics, karate, yoga, and ballet are great options to choose from. Stretching after your workout will assist you in improving your flexibility.

Conclusion

Seating at the desk or in front of the TV is never helpful for a healthy body and mind. There is more you need to know. In a nutshell, exercise is the best medicine for the body and mind. We all know that working out is not only a way of life, but it is the way we connect with ourselves, clear our minds, boost our immune system, and make time for ourselves.

I believe that exercise can be your best friend if you try hard enough. One hour in the morning or evening to yourself is extremely important. Personally, I suggest that you do it in the morning because it is the most crucial time to get yourself in shape. It is the peak time when your body burns more calories.

Outdoor exercises are more effective for the brain. The reason is fresh oxygen, more relaxing ambience, and talking to other people while exercising outdoors. I suggest that you walk at least two miles every day. You will notice the difference in your body. You will lose weight faster and healthier than you had expected. Try using weight watchers in different companies to keep track of the changes in your body. Avoid unhealthy and processed foods.

Exercise is one of the best habits that you can develop in yourself. We all need time to think and resolve all the questions we have had in our heads for a long time to get our answers and clear out our minds. We can do it all while exercising and relaxing our brain with our physical routine.

Usual issues related to aging can be resolved through exercising. However, it takes time, patience, and persistence. All of the above things we discussed do matter a great deal, as having glowing skin and a healthy body is not an overnight process. It does not happen with any miracle cures. At least, I do not know of any. I love taking care of my skin and body. I think it shows that I feel confident about myself. In the same way, my ultimate goal is to make everyone feel just as I do. I hope you stick around throughout the end of this journey so that I can share with you all my secrets to a younger, healthier skin and body.

Chapter 6- The Products

Anything good in this world does not come without any efforts. If it's easy, then you are lucky, but of course, you can't always rely on luck. If it does require a lot of your attention, then the results will definitely be worth it. When it comes to a skincare routine, there are two types of people: those who overdo it and those who underdo it. In general, females occupy the former category while males the latter, but not always. I have come across many women who did not really pay attention to their skin throughout my journey of working as an aesthetician.

However, products play a very important role in setting up your skincare routine. The right products can prove to be heaven for your skin, just as how the wrong ones can completely ruin it. Therefore, you need to be very careful about the products you choose for yourself, which is also the major reason we have a separate chapter dedicated to the products.

If you are going to choose the wrong products, it is going to have consequences. These consequences can be mild to severe, including rashes and acne. So, the next question you may ask is:

What Products Are Best for My Skin?

The ingredients on skincare products can be equivalent to reading some foreign language, except if you have a Latin background or a chemistry degree. However, manufacturers at times put a more common name in parentheses next to the scientific name, for instance, Tocopherol (Vitamin E). Without that little nudge, the list of ingredients often looks like a string of long, unfamiliar words separated by commas.

It is a lot easier to opt for a product with a cult following, especially in today's beauty influencers' age. But you should know that it's definitely not the best route. As I said earlier, there is no one-size-fits-all skincare solution. According to your needs and skin type, a customized approach is crucial to finding the right skincare products with the right ingredients for your skin. I agree that it does take a little extra time, and yes, it involves reading the ingredients list, but in the end, it sure is worth it.

Here are the dos and don'ts you should know while selecting a skincare product for yourself.

Know Your Skin Type

Your skin type is the most important factor that you need to consider while determining what skincare products will work best for you. You may know it already, but those with sensitive and acne-prone skin need to be the most cautious with different ingredients in their skincare products. However, there is good news for all those oily skin types out there. You are actually the winners here. Oily skin can handle a wider range of ingredients that can sometimes trigger irritation or breakout to other skin types.

Don't Buy into the Hype

Popularity and packaging are the easiest traps that we can all fall into, but they usually don't hold too much value or weight when it comes down to what's best for our skin. If you are going to buy something on the basis of a friend or an influencer's recommendation, then prepared to be disappointed. Instead of being influenced by how good their skin looks now, you should look out for what type of skin they were dealing with, to begin with. This will give you a clearer picture as to whether the product will work for you or not.

Natural Doesn't Always Mean Better

It can be comforting to see familiar words in the list of ingredients. However, as mentioned earlier, it sure isn't the safest route to take. According to doctors, the terms *natural* and *organic* on a product's label are more of a marketing trick than anything else. There are not any specific industry standards for them, and those terms are not regulated. They can surely offer fake promises. Moreover, sometimes a product is labeled as *natural* in reference to only one or two of the ingredients on the list.

Pay Attention to the Order of Ingredients

You will definitely want to pay attention to the list of ingredients once you know what primary ingredients you are looking to avoid or go after. It is important for you to know exactly where they fall in the ingredients list. As a good rule of thumb, Dr. David, a dermatologist, recommends that we look at the first five ingredients on the packaging since that will often account for about 80% of its makeup.

Ingredients are always listed in order of highest to lowest concentration, so if there's a problematic or potentially irritating ingredient among the first five listed, you will want to steer clear of that product. Similarly, if you seek out a product for specific ingredients, but those ingredients are listed at the end, then the product is definitely not worth your money. You will not experience many benefits of the ingredients mentioned at the end of the list since they will only be a small percentage of the overall product.

Don't Fear the Long Ingredients List

We are often taught to look for a shorter and more familiar ingredients list when it comes down to the food we put in our bodies. While a more abbreviated list can be easier to decode, it will not always cut it in terms of what you are looking to get out of your skincare products.

When you are investing in medical-grade skincare products or just looking for anti-aging properties, the ingredients list will automatically get a bit longer. It should not deter you from buying it. Instead, to help determine if the product is a good choice for you, call in for a little bit of backup, either discussing with a dermatologist or looking up the internet.

These are just a few crucial factors that you need to keep in your mind while buying skincare products.[21]

My Skincare Journey

Let's get a little personal and call it my skincare journey. There are a number of products available on the market under the title of skincare products, but what products are really good for my skin? Let's look at the harmful ingredients most skincare products contain. I can only name some of the ingredients that you avoid if you possibly can.

-   Parabens are an inexpensive and common type of preservatives used in many different skincare products to keep the product fresh

-   Sodium lauryl Sulphate

-   Petrolatum

-   Triclosan

-   Oxybenzone

---

[21]How to Choose the Skincare Products Best Suited for Your Skin, According to Dermatologists
https://www.realsimple.com/beauty-fashion/skincare/how-to-choose-skin-care-products

In my opinion, don't be afraid to use products on your skin, as long as you see no active reaction, not agreeable to your skin. When you get your hands on the good products, you will know it right away only by looking at your skin.

Sometimes, it is difficult to recognize each ingredient's name because the ingredients may be given a different name in some particular products, but the meaning of the ingredient remains the same. Let's dig in a little more and be more specific about skincare products' ingredients so that you know exactly what not to look for when opting for a product.

Benzol Alcohol

Benzyl alcohol is yet another option that is active against gram plus bacteria from 25 ppm. Generally, it is combined with acetic acid to better combat yeast and molds. Benzyl alcohol is commonly used at up to 1.0%, and acetic acid, also known as anhydrous, up to 0.6%. This mixture is safest at a PH of between 3 and 5. Incompatibility is low except with the ionic surfactants, and this combination can be obtained from nature.

Natural SLS

All skincare brands that use natural and organic high-quality ingredients in concentration to nourish skin use premium quality. Sodium lauryl sulfate serves as a cleaner. This is because they know it is gentle, safe, and effective, even on sensitive skin. Natural sodium lauryl sulfate is derived from the flesh of sustainably collected coconuts. It is important to know that it comes in seven grades, and natural skincare brands use this ingredient the most.

The cheaper and more commonly used natural alternatives to SLS such as decyl glucoside, sodium cocoyl isethionate, and sodium cocoyl glutamate, are put together in a sulfuric acid reaction. Furthermore, sodium hydroxide neutralizes it. It reacts with the natural sebum in the skin, which in turn clogs the pores. It can also bring about a burning sensation and irritate the skin, especially for those prone to acne and sensitive skin. Still, most companies use cheaper SLS because it's an inexpensive ingredient that creates a good *lather* effect.

The alternative to sodium lauryl sulfate would be ingredients that contain Vitamin E, ingredients with antiseptic properties, anti-inflammatory ingredients, hydrolyzed wheat benzoic acid, benzyl benzoate, and those high in inflammation.

Petrolatum

Petrolatum, which is another word for petroleum, is a rich moisturizer and a skin protectant approved by FDA. It is one of the most common ingredients for dry skin, including the area around the eyes, whereas refined petrolatum is approved for human usage. Most people do not know that petrolatum can actually prove to be a potentially harmful skincare product. There are risks of contamination present when using this ingredient.

This is due to the great number of cheap imitations and mass products, leading to unfavorable results. Moisturizing products such as moisturizers and lip balms contain petrolatum. However, they do not contain properties of moisturizing. Instead, it creates a barrier that keeps a hang of the moisture. It also prevents the absorption of external moisture at the same time. This suffocates the skin, and eventually, it dries out.

Petrolatum-based products act faster and give quick but temporary results. They provide a temporary illusion that your skin is soft and hydrated. I would rather not use any of these ingredients than staying in a false reality.

Hydroquinone

Hydroquinone is an aromatic compound present in skincare products and is responsible for working as a skin lightening agent. It can be helpful in the treatment of different forms of hyperpigmentation. It bleaches the skin and also decreases the number of melanocytes present in the skin. Melanocytes are the cells that form melanin, the agents responsible for producing the skin color. It helps with hyperpigmentation, which includes acne scars, age spots, freckles, melisma, and spot-inflammatory whitening of the skin because of the lack of pigment cells. However, the chemical destroys the skin when used overnight because of the lack of pigment cells, and over time, the chemical destroys the skin through its forced and harsh alteration.

This can lead to a number of skin problems, including more blemishes and even pre-aging. It is also a possible cause of a skin disease called ochronosis, where permanent patches of blue or black persist on the skin. Hydroquinone is also a possible carcinogen and may contain other toxic substances.

However, it can be used with vitamin B3 and vitamin C for more natural and safer results since it lightens the skin by daily usage.

Biotherapy Esthetics Skincare Line

When it comes to choosing the right products for yourself, you will find the best ingredients in the Biotherapy Esthetic Skincare line. Biotherapy Esthetics consists of carefully designed skincare products. Each ingredient in our product line is carefully studied and approved by myself first. This skincare line has no hazardous ingredients. They contain no artificial fragrances.

As we talked about earlier in this chapter, our product line contains no oxybenzone, petrolatum, active alcohol, or any sodium sulfate. It took me about four years to complete my product line, and it is very close to my heart. Over time, as a paramedical esthetician, with 40 years' practice of skincare treatment at my skincare clinic in San Mateo, California, I have learned a lot. I also had fellow estheticians as employees, working together to create the best experience for our clients.

With more than 1,000 repeated clients and working five to six days a week, at the end of the day, it was indeed a rewarding and pleasant experience. When I saw improvements in my clients' skin, it made me so happy. My precious and valuable clients gave me the idea of coming up with a book of my own. That's when I gave it a thought and, after some time, finally started writing a book.

Over time, I have been receiving calls from them asking about the book. They would tell me how much they liked the idea of a book out there, which would contain all the skincare knowledge that I possess. They told me how much they appreciated all the kindness I showed them. The only question they ask me whenever we converse is, *when will I be writing a book for them?*

They are truly the reason I got the confidence to write a book. They have been pushing me throughout this whole process of execution, asking me to answer all the questions as to what it takes to look younger than your actual age. They were always interested in knowing what I do to make my skin look youthful, and hence, now the secret's finally out.

I also encountered situations when young kids looked like older women, and there was no such thing as youthfulness on the faces of schoolgoing kids. Mothers with such kids would bring them to me, asking me how I could help their kids get rid of acne and enjoy clear skin so that they could continue their schooldays without losing their confidence and friends at school. It made me the happiest when I watched those kids improve and fall in love with themselves.

How I Came Up with the Idea

If I talk about how I came up with the idea of launching my skincare line and how you can treat your skin with the right products to be able to see the difference on your skin, here's a long-short story.

Over the years, I had to use different skincare lines from numerous vendors at my skincare clinic to complete my clients' treatments and help every one of them. I would suggest several different ways through which they can improve their skin and look their best. As time went by, I realized that I was never satisfied with the results. I was not receiving what I was looking for, and hence, I started spending more time finding the right products and trying out different things on each of my client's skin.

There was a time I found myself mixing ingredients of the products trying to fix the skin problem at hand. Believe me! It was working better than the line I was paying for, which was also much expensive. That's when I came up with the idea of designing my skincare line.

Using my experience with the ingredients to see results, the products that I felt were beneficial, I decided to keep them in my product line. For instance, using a certain day cream, night cream, or any piece of these positive and strong ingredients of the skincare line, I was developing my line of products over time.

Moreover, I was taking extra courses, seminars, information classes, and traveling to different states of the U.S.A. to follow up with the best of information and take classes about healthy ingredients. Some of my education classes and seminars were from Dr. Sobel in Las Vegas, Dr. Murad, Dr. Coats at Skin Esthetics school. I kept attending more and more seminars over time.

One day, I was looking at a wall in my skincare clinic. I noticed 24 skincare diplomas under my name. That's when I realized I had enough information and experience to develop a skincare line of my own. Since then, I am using my products on myself, my friends, family, and valuable clients, and I assure everyone who uses or would like to use Biotherapy Esthetics products will definitely witness the best results.

Take Care of Your Eating Habits

Eat as healthy as possible and avoid harmful ingredients. If you specifically want to benefit your skin via your eating habits, then consume vitamin-rich food. You have probably heard the saying, *you are what you eat.* So when it comes down to how well you age, this is especially true.

A huge Dutch study from 2019, in which more than 2,700 participated, concluded that dietary habits are associated with facial wrinkling, especially in women. According to the study, women whose diet includes a high amount of meat and unhealthy snacks tend to have facial wrinkles than women who include more fruits in their diet.

Foods that are high in anti-inflammatory or antioxidant properties may also improve the skin's elasticity and protect against skin damage and premature aging. Some foods and drinks with these qualities include:

- Green tea

- Olive oil

- Salmon

- Avocado

- Pomegranate

- Flax seeds

- Vegetables, especially carrots, pumpkin, leafy greens, bell peppers, and broccoli

Important Tip: DO NOT SMOKE!

I am strongly against smoking, especially when it comes to women. Cigarettes or any way through which you smoke tobacco damages collagen and elasticity of the skin. Collagen is the fiber that gives your skin the strength to maintain its youthfulness.

According to research, the heat associated with cigarettes may also cause wrinkles. Additionally, the repeated pursing of the lips to inhale may lead to premature wrinkles around the mouth. A 2013 study done on 79 pairs of identical twins found that the twins who smoked had significantly more wrinkles than their counterparts who didn't smoke.

If you currently smoke, talk to your healthcare provider about a smoking cessation program to help you quit smoking. Remember, when you are physically healthy and look good, you feel good. Wrinkles are an inevitable part of aging, but there are steps you can take to slow their progress and prevent new ones from forming.

Lifestyle factors like eating a vitamin-rich diet, drinking plenty of water, protecting your skin from the sun, not smoking, and managing your stress play a key role when it comes to keeping your skin healthy and youthful. Using retinol and a moisturizer that contains hyaluronic acid and vitamin C can also be effective at preventing the onset of wrinkles. If you have questions or concerns about products that may help prevent wrinkles, opt for the Biotherapy Skincare line and make sure to follow up with your esthetician or dermatologist.

Chapter 7- Choose the Right Skincare Products for Your Skin Daily Routine

As we talked about in the previous chapter, choosing the right products is extremely important. So what products should you use in your daily routine? What are the right steps you can take to care for your skin on a daily basis? I have said this many times previously and will say again that skin is the largest organ of your body and taking care of your skin can have a direct effect on your overall health.

Your skin acts as a protective cover for your body and is most vulnerable to the elements in the atmosphere. It is affected by more constituents than you can imagine or think of. For instance, the following factors can play a role in your skin's overall health.

- Exposure to UV radiation in tanning beds

- Exposure to chemical toxins in tobacco

- Unprotected sun exposure for long periods

- Not getting enough rest, fluid, or nutrition, which results in aging

- Drinking hard or unmoderated alcohol

Taking Care of Your Skin

It is not easy to care for your skin on a daily basis with our busy and stressful schedules. We all go through a phase when we have no attention to pay to ourselves. However, you need to take care of your skin, even if you do not have the time. Besides a daily skincare routine, make it a habit to examine your skin for abnormality, discoloration, or any other changes regularly. You must have your skin examined by a doctor or dermatologist for any changes or if:

- You have fair skin or large moles.

- You are in the sun or using tanning beds.

- You have a history of skin problems, irritations, or random growth.

It is also important to protect your skin from too much sun damage, which may add to wrinkles and result in skin cancer. Use a sunscreen or cover your skin to protect your skin from the damaging rays of the sun. If any skin irritation or problem arises, immediately see your doctor.

Understanding Skincare Products

Many products are presented as a surefire way to turn back the clock, melt away cellulite permanently, reduce wrinkles, and much more. Pay attention to them and do your research first before you decide whether a product is necessary for your skin health or is potentially harmful. Ask your doctor for advice.

As the U.S. Food and Drug Administration (FDA) regulates many products, it must regulate product instructions that change a person's physical structure or biochemical process within the body. Products that are classified as dietary supplements or cosmetics are not regulated.

Vitamins C Is Essential

I would like to explain one more product that is greatly beneficial to the skin: face powder. Using a face powder instead of liquor makeup can be very beneficial for your skin. Since vitamin C is present in it, it clears the skin, soothes it, and lightens the skin color. I can say for myself that for as long as I remember, I never used liquor makeup on my skin. I would always only use my powder. The results you can see over time are unbelievable.

Vitamin C is a necessary nutrient that has numerous functions in your body. Unlike most animals, the human body cannot make vitamin C itself. You need to get vitamin C externally and include it in your diet through foods like citrus fruit, fish, bell pepper, and leafy green. Vitamins C is particularly important for maintaining healthy-looking skin.

The reason behind this is that your skin cells use this vitamin to protect from stress caused by smoking, UV rays, and environmental pollution. In order to create collagen, our skin definitely needs vitamin C. Why is collagen so important? Because collagen is a protein that makes up more than 70% of the dry weight of your skin.

Face powder with vitamin C is a relatively new product on the market. Vitamin C acts as an antioxidant. It is the most abundant antioxidant of your skin needs. Your skin cells store vitamin C to prevent damage from environmental factors. UV rays, pollution, and smoking can all damage your skin by creating free radicals. Free radicals are unstable molecules that pull electrons from your cells and cause damage. However, vitamin C promotes collagen production, and collagen makes up the majority of the dry skin along with lightening it.

Your Diet Is Important

New research suggests that a diet high in sugar or dairy leads to a higher rate of acne. The study also found that pollution and other environmental factors might take a toll on your skin's appearance. Many have turned to strict diets for clear skin, avoiding sugar, dairy, or caffeine. However, have you ever wondered if there is any evidence that your diet will destroy your complexion or is it just another skincare myth?

Now a new study adds to mounting evidence that what you eat affects whether you break out or not. According to new research presented at this year's European Academy of Dermatology and Venereology in Madrid, researchers found that people with acne are far more likely to eat dairy products daily.

I believe there is nothing better than having a daily skincare routine to avoid skin damage. As we talked about earlier in the chapters, you can start a daily skincare routine, taking care of your skin, face, and body. Our skin surely needs help to keep us going. Here's what you can do.

Night Skin Care Routine

I will list suggest easy steps for both morning and night.

- Always at nighttime before bedtime, a strong cleanser, always with oxygen in it to be able to open the pores and exfoliating the skin, is necessary,

- After washing the skin, remove the foaming cleanser from your skin and follow with the toner (lotion) with a piece of cotton, even on your eyelids.

- To finish cleansing the skin, leave the pores ready to absorb the eye cream and follow with a night cream.

- Do not forget the neck and delicate areas. They are especially important. The neck area is very delicate. It is extremely helpful to use the eye cream on the neck, under the chin area.

- Also, try performing a different treatment every day at night. For instance, dedicate a day to help on brown spots and dryness and another night for fine wrinkles or acne.

- At night routine, before applying the night cream, it is very helpful to use a layer of glycolic acid all over the face and follow with a night cream.

Morning Skincare Routine

Our next steps come in the morning.

- Wash the skin, face and neck area. It is a wonderful idea if you use a scrub with glycolic acid.

- The time you shower is the best time to use a scrub.

- After all the skin is very clean, apply toner again.

- Eye cream, day moisturizer, and sunblock with SPF 30 are what I recommend to most clients.

- On top of the sunblock, you can apply your makeup if you must.

Makeup is extremely healthy for the skin. I always prefer face power because liquid foundation clogs the pores most of the time. Of all my years as I remember, I have never used a liquid makeup foundation.

As we are talking about a skincare routine, here is another wonderful skin treatment that you can use at least once a week. I highly recommend facial to the skin, and it is not always necessary to have a facial at the day spa. A home facial is another wonderful way the skin always benefits from.

Step 1: Wash the skin with cleanser and scrub with glycolic acid in it.

Step 2: Apply a layer of glycolic acid and eye cream around the eye.

Step 3: Apply the mask on the face and neck area. A clay mask is always the best choice. Prefer with no color or fragrance in it. The smell of the products may cause dryness or irritation to the skin. The mask has to cover the face as well as neck.

Step 4: Leave the mask on for 10 minutes.

Step 5: Remove the mask with a washcloth and warm water. The skin needs to be rinsed well from the mask impurities. Wash with water very well.

Step 6: Apply toner all over the face and neck, then eye cream, moisturizer, and night cream if it is night.

It is especially important that you opt for a facial treatment at nighttime or at the end of the day, when you know that you will not be involved in any outdoor activities. You need to be sure that you do not need any makeup application after the facial. After all the steps of a home facial are done, you will witness amazing results. It is a wonderful way to treat your skin. The skin feels soft and looks clearer and firm. Once a week, a home facial is one of the best ways to treat your skin.

Vitamin C Serum

Another wonderful ingredient that benefits your skin is vitamin C serum when it comes down to home facial treatment. Vitamin C comes in two different forms, sometimes in the form of a serum and other times in the form of cream. It is good in both ways.

So what is it about vitamin C that makes it so good? Vitamin C lightens the skin over time. It helps reduce brown spots and dark circles under the eyes. It is pretty safe to use at almost any age. The proper way to use it is every day and night under any moisturizer. It makes the skin look fresher and clearer in the daytime, which happens due to its potential anti-aging, anti-inflammatory, or muscle-building properties. Applying it at night is more beneficial for removing brown spots over time.

The Bio Peptide

Another product that I highly recommend to be used as a moisturizer is the Bio Peptide. It is a compound that firms the upper layer of the skin. It basically is a smaller version of proteins. Numerous health and cosmetics products contain different peptides for many uses, as they contain anti-inflammatory, anti-aging, and muscle-building properties. The most prominent benefit of using bio peptide is slowing down the aging process and reducing inflammation.

What is a peptide made of? Basically, it has been made from amino acids. Some of the most popular peptides include collagen peptides, which serve as an anti-aging agent and are good for the skin's overall health.

Moreover, in Biotherapy Esthetic Skincare line, you will find the face-firming complex, which is a creamy serum. It is a very effective product when it comes to firming the skin.

It is the combination of all; amino acid, peptide, and collagen.

Face-firming cream can be used again. It works best when used under the night cream. Your skin gets the opportunity to absorb it all night. It is important to be used on exceptionally clean skin. You can buy this from my website.

Chapter 8- Understand Epidermis; Skin Is the Largest Organ of the Body

Can you say that you know your skin? A lot of people do not really know their skin, especially when we get into older age. Most people do not realize that skin is an extremely important part of our body and deserves equal attention as we pay to other body parts.

When I say that skin is the largest organ of the body, I mean it. It covers a total area of about 20 square feet. The skin protects us from microbes, helps regulate body temperature, and allows the sensations of touch, heat, and cold.

Healthy Skin Begins with a Healthy Diet

A healthy diet positively affects not only your skin but also overall health. Drinking enough water can help increase your energy level and melt your fat. Moreover, stress is a common problem for a number of people.

How to Reduce Stress Level

Here are a few effective ways that can help you release anxiety and stress.

Exercise

Exercise is at number one when it comes to helping your skin look younger and healthier. In fact, it has countless health benefits. It also helps improve confidence. You may feel more competent and confident inside your body when you exercise regularly, which, in turn, promotes mental well-being.

Try to find exercises and activities that you enjoy to add to your day-to-day routines such as walking, dancing, and yoga. Activities like walking or jogging that involve repetitive movements of large muscles can particularly relieve stress. Regular exercise can help lower anxiety and stress levels by releasing endorphins and improving your sleep and self-image.

Caffeine

Caffeine is another helpful tool to reduce stress. But what is caffeine really? It is a stimulant found in tea, coffee, chocolate, and energy drinks. A high dosage may even increase anxiety. Although, a number of studies show that coffee can be healthy in moderation for everyone. In general, five or fewer cups per day is considered a moderate amount. A high quantity of caffeine can add up to the already present anxiety and stress. However, people's sensitivity to caffeine can vary greatly.

Social Support

Another wonderful way to release stress in your body is through social support from your family or friends. You may take it for granted, but it can help you in tough times. One study found that women's time spent with friends and children helps release oxytocin, a natural stress reliever. This effect is called *tend and befriend* and is the opposite of the *fight or flight* response.

Stop Procrastinating

Another way to control your stress is, staying on top of your priorities and stop procrastinating. Get in the habit of making a to-do list organized by priority. Give yourself realistic deadlines and work your way down the list. Work on the things that need to get done today and give yourself chunks of uninterrupted time, as switching between tasks or multitasking can be stressful itself.

These are just a few easy ways through which you can help your body and mind release stress. If nothing helps, try changing your surroundings and spend some time in the fresh air. I am sure you will feel better.

What Is Epidermis?

The epidermis is the thin outer layer of the skin that works to provide protection to the body and is always visible. It does not consist of any blood vessel. Therefore, it relies on the dermis, the layer of the skin underneath it, to dispose of the waste and provide access to nutrients. Since it is the outermost layer, the thickness of the epidermis varies, depending on which body part we are talking about. It is apparent through medical knowledge that the epidermis is thinnest on the eyelids.

It is specifically important to take care of the eyelids, especially if you apply eye makeup. Wash them well as part of your daily routine. Some facts that you may not know about your eyelids include: Eyelids have no pores. They lose elasticity very early on. They always need extra care.

The epidermis acts as a barrier that protects the body from harmful chemicals, ultraviolet UV radiation, and pathogens such as bacteria. Historically, it was thought that the function of the epidermis was to regulate fluid and protect the body from mechanical injury. In recent years, we have come to understand that it is a complex system that plays a key role in how the immune system communicates and targets defense.

What Illnesses and Conditions Can Affect That Layer of Your Skin?

I will name some of the conditions related to the epidermis for you to learn. The epidermis can be affected by a number of conditions and illnesses. Anything that injures or irritates your skin or sets off your immune system can negatively affect the epidermis. Infection can occur when bacterial gets into the skin through a cut or other openings.

Some common conditions that affect the skin are:

Eczema

How can you tell that someone has eczema? It causes patches of inflamed, itchy, and reddened skin. Usually, it happens when something irritates your skin, and your immune system reacts to it. Eczema affects over 30 million people in the United States, according to the National Eczema Association.

Psoriasis

Another kind of epidermis disease is psoriasis. In this condition, your immune system attacks your skin inappropriately, causing the rapid growth of skin cells. All the skin cells pile up and form a silvery, scaly area called a plaque. The skin in this area becomes very insensitive and can be painful.

Skin Cancer

These are the most common types of skin cancer.

Basal Cell Carcinoma

According to the skin cancer foundation, over four million Americans are diagnosed with it every year. It starts in the deepest part of the epidermis and rarely spreads to the other body parts. It is not usually found in areas exposed to the sun, but it is caused by UV radiation from the sun.

Malignant Melanoma

This type of skin cancer can cause melanocytes and metastasize. It grows from a mole that has been there for a long time. Many skin conditions begin in structures in the layer below the epidermis, called the dermis, and expand into the epidermis. Some of these conditions are:

Acne: According to the American Academy of Dermatology, acne is the most frequently seen skin problem in the United States. Acne takes place when the small openings in the skin, called pores, get blocked by the buildup of dead skin, dirt, bacterial, and oil.

Sebaceous Cyst: This usually develops when the opening of the sebaceous gland becomes blocked and the gland fills up with a thick liquid. They are harmless, and small cysts usually have no symptoms. They can be painful when they get huge in size.

How to Keep Your Epidermis Healthy

It is important to keep the outer layer of your skin healthy, so it can do its job of protecting your body without any hurdles. Bacteria and other harmful substances can easily get into your body and make you sick, especially when an area of your skin gets a cut or sore or breaks down. Therefore, you have to be very careful when you are met with instances where your skin is extremely vulnerable to external factors.

Wash regularly: Get rid of oil, dead cells, and bacterial that can block pores or contribute to skin breakdown.

Clean off sweat: Wash your skin well after activities that make you sweat, like sports or being out in the heat.

Always use a skincare cleanser: I will never recommend using a bar soap for washing your face. It can clog your pores. You may also experience dry skin afterward. After washing your face, I highly recommend using a moisturizer on the epidermis. It helps prevent dryness and protect your skin from the environment.

These are a few ways that you can follow to keep your epidermis healthy.

How to Take Care of Your Child's Skin

A child's skin is ten times more sensitive than that of an adult, and so it requires special care. You have to be extremely careful, especially in the first six months of a child's birth. As we talked earlier in the chapters, the skin is the largest organ of the body. The skin helps keep your temperature normal. Blood vessels near the surface of the skin allow us to have a sense of touch and find out the temperature of the body. If you get too hot or too cold, you can feel it by touching the skin. You have to pay attention to your child's skin.

Moreover, you must protect your child's skin from external factors like the sun, wind, and any dangerous environment. Their skin is much more vulnerable to environmental factors than ours.

Dangerous Environmental Factors

How can our skin be infected by dangerous environmental factors? Here are the reasons.

Air Pollution

Air pollution is a mixture of gases and solid particles in the air. Car emissions, chemicals from factories, dust, pollen, and mold spores may be suspended as particles. Ozone, a gas layer, is a major part of air pollution in big cities. When ozone forms, air pollutants become poisonous. Inhaling them can increase the chance of you having serious health problems. Air pollution is not only outside. The air inside the building can also be polluted and can affect your health in numerous ways.

Basic Toxicology

Toxicology is a branch of biology. It is basically the chemistry and medicine related to the study of the adverse effects of chemicals on living organisms. It is the study of mechanisms, symptoms, treatments, and detection of poisoning, especially the poisoning of people.

A Roman physician from the first century, also considered as the father of toxicology, is credited with the classic toxicology maxim. All things are poison, and nothing is without poison. It is only the consumption that makes something either beneficial or poisonous. This is often condensed to *the dose makes the poison.*

Chapter 9- Do You Use the Products Right?

Clear skin is a dream of every woman, but you need to make efforts to achieve that. When setting up a skincare routine, you might have an objective in mind. You can choose the products, depending on what type of results you aim to achieve. You need to be very careful of the products you use and the ingredients you put on your face.

We talked about how you can protect your skin from environmental factors in the previous chapter. However, some other ways to have clear skin are protecting it from sun damage and reducing brown spots. In order to do so, you must check the ingredients while buying products for your skin. Make sure it contains retinol, which comes in the form of a cream or serum.

What Is Retinol?

Retinol is a chemical compound that peels the skin to penetrate the third layer of the skin. Through that layer, it repairs the epidermis into clear and healthy-looking skin. In simpler words, retinol sinks into your skin and speeds up cell turnover, causing your body to churn out fresher, smoother skin once again. This is the reason why it is mostly present in anti-aging creams. Now, let's look at what basic characteristics an ideal retinol cream should have.

Analysis

Ideal retinol cream is loaded with all the ingredients that can balance out the effect of this chemical. BioCare offers the most effective retinol cream that we have personally tried out. It contains 0.5% retinol that sets it apart from all other products in this category. Encapsulated retinol works similar to regular retinol. However, it delivers its power into the skin differently.

Retinol has been housed in a carrier system to protect its integrity and improve its ability to penetrate the skin effectively. The retinol cream also contains the ingredient *ceramides* to restore moisture into the skin.

Usage

You have to be very careful about the consistency of using retinol. It is best to use it for one week and then stop for two weeks, and then start it again. The best time to use it is the nighttime after cleansing the skin with toner.

Using retinol for a long time can make the first layer of the skin very thin and sensitive. It is why it is not recommended to be used over a long period of time. You must always wash off retinol in the morning with a soft cleanser.

Vitamin C Powder

Another ingredient that can prove to be very effective for your skin is vitamin C powder. There are a lot of benefits of applying vitamin C to your skin. Let's look at a few of them.

-   In order to prevent the damage from environmental factors, your skin cells store vitamin C. UV rays, pollution, and smoking can all damage your skin by creating free radicals. Vitamin C can help repair that damage.

-   Vitamin C promotes collagen production, and collagen makes up the majority of the dry weight of your skin. In order to synthesize this protein, your body needs vitamin C. Many of the symptoms of vitamin C deficiency are caused by impaired collagen synthesis.

- Vitamin C lightens skin color.

- Oftentimes, vitamin C can prove to be a solution to treat sun damage.

These are just a few reasons of how beneficial vitamin C can prove to be for your skin. It can be used in a few different forms, as a day moisturizer, as a night serum, or as a face mask.

Usage

I discovered the benefits of this amazing ingredient when I began to use the vitamin C mask at least once a week. The results left me astonished, and my skin responded wonderfully to it.

Vitamin C always comes in the form of powder. You can mix it with warm water until it forms a paste that's consistent enough to be applied to the skin.

Apply it over your face and avoid the area around your eyes. It is best to apply it over the neck area. Leave the mask on for at least 10 minutes. After that, wash it off with warm water using a sponge or washcloth. Follow up with toner, vitamin C serum, and moisturizer.

Remember that whatever you are applying over your skin, it is best to use it at night. This is because it is when your skin and blood circulation are resting, which is the best condition for the product to penetrate through the pores and into the third layers of the skin.

In this chapter, I am going to explain numerous ways through which you can achieve the goal of healthy skin. Right now, I am taking a break to give you some quick tips for healthy skin.

- Protect your skin from the sun.

- Don't smoke.

- Treat your skin gently.

- Eat a healthy diet.

- Manage stress.

- Set up a good skincare routine - sun protection, a strong cleanser, day moisturizer, night cream, and under-eye cream can keep your skin healthy and glowing.

Let's talk about another major problem that we face as we age, which is wrinkles. Some natural wrinkles look good on our faces, but not all of them. Let's first find this out.

What Causes Wrinkles?

Everyone wants to slow down the process of aging, and since wrinkles are one of the signs of aging, they must be worked upon. There is no harm in having wrinkles. A few facial lines can be endearing and add character to your face. However, it is no secret that many of us prefer to keep them in check.

Once you have them, it can be challenging to reverse the appearance of wrinkles, especially without medical or surgical intervention. But there are steps that you can take to help reduce them. In fact, you can easily make a few lifestyle changes to slow down their appearance.

What Can You Do to Prevent Wrinkles?

Genetics plays a major role in how you age as time passes. But even if your family has a skin history that tends to wrinkle easily, you can have a good deal of control over your skin and how well it ages.

When you take good care of your skin, it can go a long way in keeping your skin wrinkle-free for as long as possible, although it is inevitable that wrinkles will show up at some point in life.

Here are a few steps you can take to prevent wrinkles.

- As I explained in the chapters earlier, a healthy diet and proper skin care regimen can go a long way in keeping your skin healthy and young.

- Always protect your skin from the sun.

- Always apply a moisturizer over your skin.

- Smoking and alcohol are the worst enemies of your skin and body. Please don't do it.

- Do not forget to take your vitamins.

According to a huge Dutch study from 2019, more than 2,700 people participated and found that our eating habits are associated with our facial wrinkling, especially in women. The study concluded that the women whose diets include a higher ratio of red meat and unhealthy snacks tend to have more facial wrinkles than the women who include more fruits, vegetables, and nutrition in their diet.

Food that is high in anti-inflammatory or antioxidant properties may also improve the skin's elasticity and prevent skin damage and premature aging. Some foods and drinks with these qualities include:

- Olive oil

- Green tea

- Salmon avocados

- Flax seeds

- Pomegranate

- Vegetables, especially carrots, pumpkins, leafy greens, bell peppers, and broccoli

Why Do We Have Wrinkles?

Wrinkles usually occur when your skin loses collagen over time. These are fibers that make your skin supple and firm. As you age, collagen losses occur naturally, and you have no control over it. But there are also a number of other skin components and certain lifestyle habits that add up to this process.

The resulting wrinkles tend to be the most noteworthy around thinner areas of your face. The good news is that you may even be able to take steps to prevent mouth wrinkles from developing prematurely, including their appearance.

Causes of Mouth Wrinkles

The area around your mouth area is one of the first spots on your face that is most likely to develop wrinkles. One of the reasons behind this is the thinness of the skin in this particular area, which already has less collagen than other areas of the face. Once you turn 20 years old, your skin starts producing an estimated 1% less collagen every year.

Other characteristics of the skin's aging process to consider besides collagen, such as a loss of elastin and glycosaminoglycan, contribute to the skin's elasticity and hydration. These are known as intrinsic or natural aging.

How to Get Rid of Wrinkles

There are many natural ways to get rid of wrinkles, but that process can be extremely slow. You can get rid of the wrinkles around your mouth and chin more quickly by using medical and aesthetics treatments.

Anti-Aging Chemical Treatment

Dermatologists may recommend you one of the most used anti-aging treatments. A chemical peel works by removing the upper layer (epidermis) of your skin to reveal smoother and radiant skin underneath. This is typically done on a monthly basis to help maintain your results.

Dermabrasion Treatment

Moreover, dermabrasion treatment can help a lot. The dermabrasion treatment is an exfoliating technique that can be used to reduce the appearance of fine wrinkles around the mouth. It is a stronger chemical treatment recommended by estheticians to remove the outer layer and up to several layers of the skin. The same treatment can be used on the entire face, neck, and delicate areas of your face.

Micro-Needling or Collagen Induction Therapy

Another treatment, micro-needling, also known as collagen induction therapy, is a procedure that uses small needles to prick your skin via a device called a derma roller or micro-needling pen. The idea is that your skin will be smoother once it heels from the small wounds made during the process. You need multiple sessions over the course of several months for the best results. The plastic surgeon or dermatologist can give the following treatment.

Dermal Fillers

There is another wonderful treatment that can be used. I call it *derma fillers*. A dermatologist or plastic surgeon might recommend injectable dermal fillers for a deeper smile and marionette lines. These are put together with ingredients like hyaluronic acid and Poly-L-Lastic acid, which help to plump the skin's targeted area to smooth out wrinkles temporarily. Derma fillers wear off after several months, and you will need to get more injections over time to help maintain results.

Botox

Administered by injections, botox works by relaxing facial muscles that might produce a tight, wrinkled appearance. It may also benefit lines in the lip and upper lip areas and refine the appearance of marionette lines, even though this treatment is best known for eye wrinkles.

Face Lift

A cosmetic surgeon may recommend a facelift to other areas that may not respond well to other treatments. This procedure helps smooth wrinkles and correct the sagging of skin via an incision, fat transfer, and the lifting of muscles and tissues, like other cosmetic surgeries. A facelift is considered a major procedure.

A Good Skincare Regiment

There are other ways to prevent wrinkles in the upper lip area and to the entire face, excluding medical interference. A good skincare regiment goes a long way in preventing the onset of premature wrinkles. Make sure you wash your face twice a day and follow up with a moisturizer and an anti-aging serum tailored to your skin type. Exfoliate at least twice a week to get rid of dead cells that make any fine lines and wrinkles disappear.

Using wrinkle products at home can help, but you may not see the results for up to some weeks. Especially for a new product to work, it may require a lot of time before you finally see the results. Some preventive measures can also go a long way in preventing wrinkles, especially around the mouth.

Taking care of your health can do wonders for your body and skin. This is why I emphasize developing healthy habits so much in each of my chapters. For best results in skincare products, I highly recommend you to visit biotherapyesthetics.com. All the products available on this website are made closely under my supervision, and I can guarantee amazing results. Believe me! You will fall in love with all the products, your skin, and yourself all over again.

Chapter 10- Type of Skin Acne and How to Treat Any Type of Acne?

Almost every one of us has experienced acne at some point in life, and it is not at all pleasant to watch your skin worsen with each passing day. It even puts some people in an inferiority complex, and they often lose confidence to go out and meet people because they constantly feel that they don't look good enough. It becomes so severe at some point that people start to believe that they will have to live with this skin for the rest of their lives. So, if you are someone who struggles with acne, relax. By the end of this chapter, you will know enough about acne to treat it the right way.

Acne is a skin condition that can occur to anyone at any age. Commonly, it tends to start at puberty, and most people experience it during this time before it resolves itself in the late teens or early 20s. However, it can persist into the late 20s and even 30s for some people.

Its severity can differ from just a few spots to larger clusters of affected areas. Acne may also appear on the back as well as face, neck, and chest. It can leave dark spots and permanent scars on the skin if left untreated. It is usually associated with hormonal fluctuations experienced during the teenage years, but adults can also experience it. As many as 17 million Americans have acne, it makes it one of the most common skin conditions among both children and adults.

However, technology has made it much easier to identify what type of acne you have. Once identified, you can look for ways through which you can heal it. You need to get to the root cause in order to find the best solution according to your skin type.

Subtypes of Acne

Acne may be inflammatory or non-inflammatory. Subtypes of acne include:

- Whiteheads

- Blackheads

- Papules

- Nodules

- Cysts

It is possible to have multiple types of acne at once. In some cases, it may even be severe enough to warrant a visit to the dermatologist. You may often hear the term *breakout* used to describe all acne forms, but this is not always a precise description. Not all types of acne grow across the skin. Clogged pores can also be the reason behind your acne. These may be attributed to:

- Excess production of oil (Sebum)

- Bacterial

- Hormones

- Dead skin cells

- Ingrown hair

The key to a successful treatment is identifying what type of acne you are experiencing. Let's look at the several types of acne in depth.

Papules

Papules acne occurs when the walls surrounding the pores of your skin break down from serious inflammation. As a result, they form hard, clogged pores that are tender to even touch. The skin around these pores is usually pink. Papules are small and usually less than a centimeter in size. They can appear in a variety of sizes, colors, and shapes.

Papules are sometimes called skin lesions, which are primarily changes in your skin color and texture. Papules often cluster together to form a rash. Most of the time, it's not something serious. In fact, it can be relieved with home treatments, depending on the cause.

Cysts

A cyst is a sac-like pocket of membranous tissue that contains air, fluid, or other substances. It can grow almost anywhere in your body or under your skin. It can develop when pores are clogged by a combination of bacteria, sebum, and dead cells. The clog occurs deep within the skin and is further beneath the surface than nodules.

These large white or red bumps are often painful to touch. Cysts are the largest form of acne. Their formation usually results from a severe infection. This type of acne is most likely to leave scars behind. In some cases, an appointment with an esthetician can give you good results, but if the acne is way too over the head, then treatment from a dermatologist may help.

How to Avoid Cysts

To avoid such acne, I highly recommend keeping the skin bacteria-free and clear of dead cells. You can do this by washing your face with a strong cleanser in the morning and at night.

Non-inflammatory Acne

This type of acne includes blackheads and whiteheads. These normally do not cause swelling. They respond relatively well to over-the-counter (OTC) treatments. I highly recommend Biotherapy Esthetic Glycolic acid for such type of acne since this acid naturally exfoliates the skin, removing dead cells that can lead to blackheads and whiteheads. Look for it in cleansers, toners, and oil-free moisturizers.

Blackheads (open pores)

Blackheads occur when a pore is clogged. This results in a characteristically black color that can be seen on the surface of the skin. This type of acne also forms when a pore gets clogged by sebum and dead skin cells, but unlike with blackheads, the top of the pore closes up. It looks like a small bump is protruding from the skin.

Whiteheads

Whiteheads occur the same way as blackheads do. The only difference is that they are even more difficult to treat because the pores are already closed.

Treatment

Products containing salicylic acid can be helpful. There is a high chance that you have already used salicylic acid in your past to treat acne. It is present in every kind of treatment these days, from lotions to cleansers. Topical retinoid gives the best results for common acne. Pimples that are swollen and red are referred to as inflammatory acne. Although dead skin cells and sebum contribute to this, bacteria can also play a role in clogging pores. The bacterium can even cause an infection deep beneath your skin's surface. This may result in painful acne spots that are difficult to get rid of.

Products containing benzoyl peroxide may help lessen swelling and get rid of bacterial in your skin. Other than that, your doctor can prescribe either an oral or topical antibiotic along with benzoyl-peroxide to treat the inflammatory acne. Topical products with retinoids are an important part of combatting the following types of acne.

How Severe Is Each Type of Acne?

Whiteheads and blackheads are the mildest forms of acne. They can sometimes be cleared up with topical medication or strong skincare products. Due to my skincare practice experience over the years, I believe that a good healthy skincare routine in your teenage years can help you avoid acne.

Cheap skincare products cause a lot of skin problems over time. Acne is an extremely uncomfortable disease, especially for our appearance. It is important to take care of our skin from the early years. Set up a good healthy diet, a skincare line of products, and stick to the morning and night routine.

How Can You Avoid Acne?

Glycolic acid is important. Do not forget to apply an oil-free moisturizer on top of glycolic acid. It may help best if you add this to your daily routine. Moreover, it really is important to note that while some treatments may work immediately, you must be patient with your acne treatment. You may not see improvement for several months. However, you should also use caution in using too many acne products at once. This can result in dry skin. In response, your pores can create more sebum. This can lead to even more acne issues. You should also confirm whether any bumps or swelling in your skin are actually acne results. Several skin conditions cause symptoms like those with acne, even though they are something entirely different.

Back Acne

Often large and tender cysts can develop on the back. These may either burst or heal up without rupturing. The area affected by the acne may feel hot, tender to the touch, or be painful. The severity of back acne can vary. Grade 1, or mild acne, usually consists of a few blemishes and may include blackheads, whiteheads, and pimples. Grade 4 acne is severe and characterized by many cysts and spots.

What Causes Back Acne?

There are numerous reasons why people get back acne, so it's important to know why and how pimples form. Your body produces an oil called sebum. It's made in the glands connected to your hair follicles. The sebum moves up the follicles to add moisture to your skin hair. Pimples form when extra sebum and dead cells skin builds up. This build-up blocks skin pores and bacteria. As a result, the hair follicle swells out and forms a whitehead pimple. When the clogged pore gets exposed to air, it forms blackhead pimples.

Treatment For Back Acne

In most cases, you can get rid of acne by making some small yet effective lifestyle changes. You can also use home remedies to get them off your back. Here are some things you can do to get rid of back acne.

Shower after a workout: Letting the sweat and dirt sit on your skin after a workout can be a huge contributor to back acne. Hence, shower as soon as you can after a workout. You should also wash those sweaty workout clothes between sweat sessions.

A strong exfoliating scrub: Use a strong exfoliating scrub with ingredients such as salicylic acid or glycolic acid. I highly recommend glycolic acid in my experience with back acne treatment, as it helps best and leaves the skin without any redness or irritation.

See a dermatologist: When nothing works for you, go and see a dermatologist. They can help you get rid of back acne with the right medications.

Home remedies: Acne is a very difficult disease to get rid of. Since most of the acne occurs due to clogged pores, it is necessary to exfoliate the skin with a strong scrub, glycolic acid, and an oil-free moisturizer. Applying aloe vera gel after washing the skin may also help.

No matter how old we are, acne is not a matter of age. When you are a teenager, getting acne is basically a rite of passage, but that does not mean the skin condition goes away when you get older. According to the American Academy of Dermatologists, 85% of people between the age of 12 and 24 experience at least minor acne.

Reasons behind Acne on Different Parts of Body

Acne is totally normal, but that does not mean it's not trying to tell you that something else is going on with your body health. There are so many reasons people get breakouts. That's why it is important to pay attention to what kind of acne you are dealing with and where you are usually breaking out.

Getting pimples on your forehead, nose, or even back can all point to different health concerns. Acne can definitely show you other health issues you may not know you are dealing with. Acne on your chin or jawline usually points to a hormonal imbalance.

According to the American Academy of Dermatology, up to 15% of women said that they struggle with hormonal acne more than men, which usually appears on the chin or jawline. So, if you have breakouts along your jawline or on your chin more than anywhere else, you may have a hormonal imbalance.

How To Prevent Facial Acne?

As I said earlier in the chapters, cleansing your skin or exfoliating your skin with the scrub is extremely important. You must do these steps every day in the morning and at night. After you are done washing, dry out with a soft towel.

When your skin dries out, use a small amount of glycolic acid gel. It has a strong effect on your skin; hence you must apply it all over the face except the area around your eyes. Allow the gel to dry and apply an oil-free moisturizer.

Applying non-comedogenic moisturizer or oil-free is best for areas with acne and the entire face. It is necessary to use SPF protection. The sun is a major source of causing brown spots. However, the skin becomes very vulnerable after all this treatment, and it becomes very difficult to get rid of the spots. Please do not forget to use sunblock on a regular basis, even on rainy days.

Topical Retinoid

Topical retinoid is another acne treatment with scar-smoothing benefits. What is a topical retinoid? Topical retinoids are creams, gels, and lotions containing medicine obtained from vitamin A. These compounds result in reduced keratinization and proliferation of skin cells, independent of their functions as a vitamin.

According to a recent review, in addition to speeding up your cell regeneration and improving your skin texture, retinoids can also help reduce discoloration and make scars less noticeable. However, they can also make your skin exceptionally sensitive to the sun, as mentioned earlier. Always remember to wear your sunblock and a moisturizer on. For skin with acne, number 30 SPF is enough because a higher number may make you feel that the acne is returning.

Dermabrasion

Dermabrasion is an exfoliating method that uses a rotating instrument to remove your skin's outer layers, usually on the face. This treatment is popular among people who wish to improve the appearance of their skin. Some of the conditions it can treat include sun damage, fine lines, uneven texture, and acne scars.

Dermabrasion is known as one of the most effective and common treatments for facial scars. You can do it at home. It uses the same general principle as the microdermabrasion kits. Healthcare providers use a wire brush or a wheel to exfoliate the layers of the skin more deeply. It is best for scars; nevertheless, deeper scars may also become less noticeable.

Fillers

Fillers are the most common treatment of our time. Dermal fillers are gel-like substances that are injected beneath the skin to restore lost volume, soften creases, and smooth lines or enhance facial contours. More than one million men and women choose this popular facial rejuvenation treatment every year, which can be a cost-effective way to look younger without surgery or downtime.

When it comes to acne scars, healthcare providers use fillers to fill in the scars, also aiding in evening out the skin. The fillers can help to plump up and smooth out depressed scars. Most fillers last six to eight months before they need to be redone, but some are permanent. This treatment is best for someone with a small number of rolling or box scars.

The Takeaway

Acne scars can be frustrating. It is like a double punishment. First, you had to deal with the pimple, and now you have scars to remind you that they were there. This is the reason why I encourage a healthy skincare routine from the very beginning. I am not saying it will prevent you from acne. I am only saying that it can help a lot in the long run.

Even if you have caught acne scars, you don't have to panic. There are a number of treatments that can make them less noticeable. A healthcare provider can help you find the perfect treatment to help reduce your scars' appearance, even though most scars are permanent.

The best way to treat acne scars is to prevent them in the first place. You are more likely to develop acne scars if you are out less. Do not touch your face often, particularly when you're out. Avoid popping, picking, or squeezing any breakout, no matter how tempting it may look. This step is important to prevent skin irritation. It is how you can save the underlying tissue from being damaged. Otherwise, it will lead to permanent scars.

Conclusion

"Live fast, die young, and leave a good looking corpse."
-John Derek

I feel proud to have finished my dream book, lend a helping hand to others struggling with skincare issues, and make a substantial difference in people's life. If you are still reading this, congratulations because you care about yourself and your skin enough to hold on till the end. The core message of this book was not only to set up a skincare routine but also to follow that routine with persistence. Therefore, I urge you to follow a skincare routine religiously to see a substantial difference in your skin.

If I reflect upon my life, a major chunk of it has always been about skincare. I have studied and practiced skincare for over 40 years, and I am more than proud of myself for being able to come up with my skincare line called the Biotherapy Esthetics. Each product under this skincare line is really close to my heart because I have picked each ingredient in it after thorough research and experience. All the products have been tested and studied closely with the help of my team of experts.

As an esthetician, I have come across many patients belonging to different age groups who suffered from skin problems. Although I helped them as much as I could, I realized how prevention would have been a much better choice for them. They would not be there sitting in my clinic due to self-confidence issues if they had taken the right steps at the right time.

This is why I believe that skincare is not only for women but also for men. As stated in the previous chapter, a good skincare routine and healthy lifestyle choices can help slow down the aging process and protect you from various skin problems. Before you go out and buy products for your skin, you need to:

Know Your Skin

Ask yourself, do you really know your skin type? You may suspect that you have oily, sensitive, or dry skin, but what next? How do you find out what's best for your skin type? When you know your skin type, it can help you buy the right cosmetics. Why is it so important to know your skin type? It is because wrong products and even popularized skin hacks can worsen dryness, acne, or any other skin problems if they are not made for your skin type.

Once you know your skin, you can easily set up a skincare routine. But no matter what your skin type is, a daily skincare routine can help you maintain overall skin health, improving scars, dark spots, and acne.

Just a reminder for you all that a good skincare routine involves five basic steps. These steps can be followed in the morning and before bed. These include a cleanser, serum, toner, moisturizer, and a good sunblock.

Remember to choose the products that fit your skin type and sensitivity. Remember to read the label before you put a product in your basket. Some products such as retinol or prescription retinoids should only be applied at night. Begin with a basic and simple routine to see how your skin reacts to it. Once your skin becomes accustomed to it, you can add extra products such as masks, exfoliants, and spot treatments to give a boost to your skin's health.

When Trying a New Product

When trying new products, don't forget to patch test, especially if you suspect that you have sensitive skin. It will help you identify potential allergic reactions if any. Follow the steps below to patch test a new product.

Apply a small amount of the product you want to test over your skin in a discreet area. For instance, try it on the side of your face close to the area near your ear and wait for 20 minutes. Then wash your skin with cold water. Check that specific area afterward to see if your skin has caught any delayed reaction or not.

Remember that an allergic reaction may include redness, irritation, itchiness, or small bumps. If you notice any of these symptoms, wash the tested area immediately with water and a cleanser. Do not use that product again, and try a different one.

Be Careful of What You Put inside Your Body

We all have a favorite face cream or a treatment we love, but the journey of beautiful skin begins with nourishment from within. Our skin cells are continually shedding and are being replaced by younger ones. A constant supply of key nutrients is necessary to support this rapid growth. When you eat the correct balance of foods and provide your skin with the vital nutrients, it helps it stay supple, blemish-free, soft, and young.

There is no denying the fact that our skin does naturally age. Aging spots and wrinkles are the inevitable results of time. However, there may be some factors speeding up the process of aging without you knowing. Tanning beds, overexposure to the sun, strong chemicals, soaps, and poor nutrition could be a few of the many reasons behind the quick aging of your skin. SA holistic approach is always best with all these factors in mind.

Treat your skin kindly, and optimize your nutrition by eating antioxidant-rich fruits and vegetables. Gain healthy fats from nuts and oily fish and try to feed yourself on a varied yet balanced diet. This should give your skin the optimal level of the crucial nutrients for radiant skin, including the necessary vitamins C and E, beta carotene, selenium, and zinc.

Time to Wrap Up

In the end, I would only say that I cannot express how happy I am to have completed my dream book. It sure is an accomplishment for me. The main purpose of this book is to help others. I really hope this book helps everyone who aims to achieve the target of healthy and younger-looking skin. I wanted to share the secret to younger-looking skin for which you must adopt a healthy lifestyle.

I am overwhelmed with joy and gratitude to say that it has been extremely rewarding for me to share my experiences. I have practiced skincare treatment for a considerably long period, and it has enabled me to help countless patients with acne and other skin problems. After all the extensive experiences I've had, I hope I have contributed to my patients' lives constructively.

In this book, in each and every chapter, I have focused on the importance of skincare. I aimed to lay out all the information I could for you to understand how you can improve your life by developing simple habits. I want people to hear questions like *What's the secret behind your amazing skin?* rather than *What happened to your face?* I really hope I was able to pull that off, and I am glad that I tried my best.

Since this book is all about healthy-looking skin, I want to leave you all with some helpful tips.

- Set up a skincare regimen for morning and night. (if you haven't already)

- Use skincare products with high-quality ingredients.

- Protect your skin from the sun.

- Apply sunblock, even on rainy days.

- Avoid alcohol.

- Eat healthy, which means avoid fatty food.

- Exercise at least three times a week.

- Please do not smoke, and teach your children not to smoke.

Taking care of ourselves is worthwhile for numerous reasons. Its effects can only be seen with time. But for time to bring change into effect, you must start altering your lifestyle, aligning it with a healthier one. Life is precious, so make sure you spend your time being the best version of yourself. Regardless of how your day is going, one positive expression can make you feel good. Try helping others. It will make you feel good about yourself.

If you are thinking of upgrading your skincare line, I highly recommend these gem of products, which you can easily get from Biotherapyethetics.com. This skincare line contains some extremely high-quality ingredients and will sure give you amazing results. Yes, you will fall in love with yourself and your skin all over again. The products include:

- Eye cream

- Super-firming cream for night

- Herbal silk day moisturizer

- Peptide serum

- Silk amino mask

There are many amazing products that you can find on my website www.biotherapyesthetics.com. Do remember to check them out and benefit from them in the long run. I will wrap up my dream book with this one motivational line for you all.

Look good. It feels good!

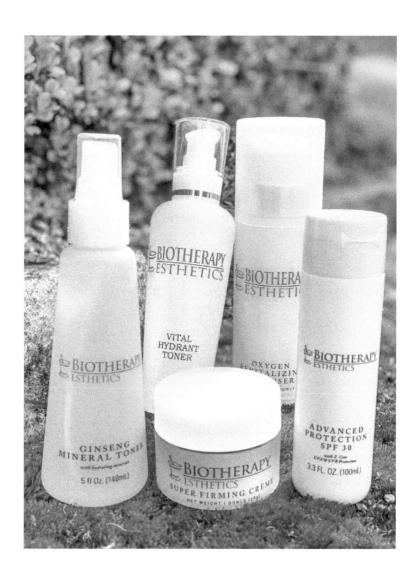

Bibliography

7 REASONS WHY YOUR SKINCARE ROUTINE IS IMPORTANT https://www.stockpilingmoms.com/7-reasons-why-your-skin-care-routine-is-important/

See study from McMaster University in Ontario: https://www.ncbi.nlm.nih.gov/pmc/articles/PMC4531076/

Glycemic index https://en.wikipedia.org/wiki/Glycemic_index

Does Drinking Water Really Make Your Skin Glow? https://thecoldestwater.com/does-drinking-water-really-make-your-skin-glow/

Your lifestyle and your skin https://www.health24.com/Lifestyle/Perfect-Skin/Natural-Beauty/Your-lifestyle-and-your-skin-20140115

Medicines and side effects https://www.betterhealth.vic.gov.au/health/ConditionsAndTreatments/medicines-and-side-effects

Why consistency is key in a skincare regime
https://my.lumitylife.com/why-consistency-is-key-in-a-skincare-regime/

This is how long it will take for your skincare routine to work https://globalnews.ca/news/4113894/skincare-routine-effects-time/

Why Is Skin Care So Important?
https://www.halecosmeceuticals.com/why-is-skin-care-so-important/

8 IMPORTANT REASONS TO PROTECT YOUR SKIN IN THE SUN https://www.timelessha.com/blogs/news/8-important-reasons-to-protect-your-skin-in-the-sun

Protecting Your Skin from the Sun https://www.cancer.net/navigating-cancer-care/prevention-and-healthy-living/protecting-your-skin-sun

Why sun protection is important https://www.reidhealth.org/blog/why-sun-protection-is-important

What Does SPF Stand For?https://www.consumerreports.org/cro/magazine/

2015/05/what-does-spf-stand-for/index.htm#:~:text=SPF%20(sun%20protection%20factor)%20is,ultraviolet%20(UV)%20B%20rays.&text=Assuming%20you%20use%20it%20correctly,protects%20for%20about%2010%20hours

WHAT IS SPF SUNSCREEN?

https://www.badgerbalm.com/s-30-what-is-spf-sunscreen-sun-protection-factor.aspx

https://www.medicalnewstoday.com/articles/318290#Twelve-myths-about-sunscreen

https://www.madesafe.org/education/whats-in-that/sunscreen/

https://theeverygirl.com/the-best-non-toxic-sunscreens/

Exercise: 7 benefits of regular physical activity
https://www.mayoclinic.org/healthy-lifestyle/fitness/in-depth/exercise/art-20048389

The Top 10 Benefits of Regular Exercise
https://www.healthline.com/nutrition/10-benefits-of-exercise#TOC_TITLE_HDR_2

The Top 10 Benefits of Regular Exercise
https://www.healthline.com/nutrition/10-benefits-of-exercise#TOC_TITLE_HDR_11

How to Choose the Skincare Products Best Suited for

Your Skin, According to Dermatologists

https://www.realsimple.com/beauty-

fashion/skincare/how-to-choose-skin-care-products

9 781801 281218